CHILDHOOD CANCER
SURVIVORSHIP

IMPROVING CARE AND QUALITY OF LIFE

National Cancer Policy Board

Maria Hewitt, Susan L. Weiner, and Joseph V. Simone, Editors

INSTITUTE OF MEDICINE
NATIONAL RESEARCH COUNCIL
OF THE NATIONAL ACADEMIES

THE NATIONAL ACADEMIES PRESS   500 Fifth Street, N.W.   Washington, DC 20001

NOTICE: The project that is the subject of this report was approved by the Governing Board of the National Research Council, whose members are drawn from the councils of the National Academy of Sciences, the National Academy of Engineering, and the Institute of Medicine. The members of the committee responsible for the report were chosen for their special competences and with regard for appropriate balance.

This study was supported by the National Cancer Institute; the Centers for Disease Control and Prevention; the American Cancer Society; Abbott Laboratories; the American Society of Clinical Oncology; Amgen, Inc.; Aventis; and the United Health Care Foundation. Any opinions, findings, conclusions, or recommendations expressed in this publication are those of the author(s) and do not necessarily reflect the views of the organizations or agencies that provided support for the project.

Library of Congress Cataloging-in-Publication Data

National Cancer Policy Board (U.S.)
  Childhood cancer survivorship : improving care and quality of life / National Cancer Policy Board ; Susan L. Weiner, Joseph V. Simone, and Maria Hewitt, editors ; Institute of Medicine and National Research Council.
      p. ; cm.
Includes bibliographical references.
  ISBN 0-309-08898-4 (pbk.) — ISBN 0-309-50581-X (PDF)
  1. Tumors in children—Complications. 2. Tumors in children—Patients—Services for. 3. Tumors in children—Government policy—United States.
  [DNLM: 1. Neoplasms—Child. 2. Survivors. 3. Follow-Up Studies. 4. Health Policy. 5. Needs Assessment. QZ 275 N277c 2003] I. Weiner, Susan Lipschitz, 1942- II. Simone, Joseph V. III. Hewitt, Maria Elizabeth. IV. Title.
  RC281.C4N367 2003
  362.1'9892994—dc21

                              2003008030

Additional copies of this report are available from the National Academies Press, 500 Fifth Street, N.W., Lockbox 285, Washington, DC 20055; (800) 624-6242 or (202) 334-3313 (in the Washington metropolitan area); Internet, http://www.nap.edu

COVER: Candlelighters Childhood Cancer Foundation, National Office; Candlelighters of the El Paso Area Inc., and Sunset Color Graphics, El Paso (photographer).

THE NATIONAL ACADEMIES
Advisers to the Nation on Science, Engineering, and Medicine

The **National Academy of Sciences** is a private, nonprofit, self-perpetuating society of distinguished scholars engaged in scientific and engineering research, dedicated to the furtherance of science and technology and to their use for the general welfare. Upon the authority of the charter granted to it by the Congress in 1863, the Academy has a mandate that requires it to advise the federal government on scientific and technical matters. Dr. Bruce M. Alberts is president of the National Academy of Sciences.

The **National Academy of Engineering** was established in 1964, under the charter of the National Academy of Sciences, as a parallel organization of outstanding engineers. It is autonomous in its administration and in the selection of its members, sharing with the National Academy of Sciences the responsibility for advising the federal government. The National Academy of Engineering also sponsors engineering programs aimed at meeting national needs, encourages education and research, and recognizes the superior achievements of engineers. Dr. Wm. A. Wulf is president of the National Academy of Engineering.

The **Institute of Medicine** was established in 1970 by the National Academy of Sciences to secure the services of eminent members of appropriate professions in the examination of policy matters pertaining to the health of the public. The Institute acts under the responsibility given to the National Academy of Sciences by its congressional charter to be an adviser to the federal government and, upon its own initiative, to identify issues of medical care, research, and education. Dr. Harvey V. Fineberg is president of the Institute of Medicine.

The **National Research Council** was organized by the National Academy of Sciences in 1916 to associate the broad community of science and technology with the Academy's purposes of furthering knowledge and advising the federal government. Functioning in accordance with general policies determined by the Academy, the Council has become the principal operating agency of both the National Academy of Sciences and the National Academy of Engineering in providing services to the government, the public, and the scientific and engineering communities. The Council is administered jointly by both Academies and the Institute of Medicine. Dr. Bruce M. Alberts and Dr. Wm. A. Wulf are chair and vice chair, respectively, of the National Research Council.

www.national-academies.org

PILAR OSSORIO, Assistant Professor of Law & Medical Ethics, Associate Director for Programming, Center for the Study of Race and Ethnicity in Medicine, University of Wisconsin Law School, Madison, WI (member through April 2002)

CECIL B. PICKETT, Executive Vice President, Discovery Research, Schering-Plough Research Institute, Kenilworth, NJ

LOUISE RUSSELL, Professor, Rutgers University, New Brunswick, NJ

JOHN SEFFRIN, Chief Executive Officer, American Cancer Society, Atlanta, GA (member through April 2002)

THOMAS J. SMITH, Professor, Virginia Commonwealth University, Richmond, VA

SANDRA UNDERWOOD, ACS Oncology Nursing Professor, University of Wisconsin School of Nursing, Milwaukee, WI (member through April 2002)

SUSAN WEINER, President, The Children's Cause, Silver Spring, MD

ROBERT C. YOUNG, President, American Cancer Society and the Fox Chase Cancer Center, Philadelphia, PA

Consultants

F. Daniel Armstrong, PhD, University of Miami School of Medicine

Alice G. Ettinger, RN, MSN, St. Peter's University Hospital, New Brunswick, NJ

Daniel Green, MD, Roswell Park Cancer Institute, Buffalo, NY

Anna T. Meadows, MD, The Children's Hospital of Philadelphia

Raymond Mulhern, PhD, St. Jude Children's Research Hospital and University of Tennessee College of Medicine

Sharon Murphy, MD, Children's Memorial Hospital, Chicago

Kevin Oeffinger, MD University of Texas Southwestern Medical Center at Dallas

Leslie Robison, PhD, University of Minnesota Cancer Center

Brad Zebrack, PhD, MSW, David Geffen School of Medicine at UCLA, Los Angeles, CA

Lonnie Zeltzer, MD, David Geffen School of Medicine at UCLA, Los Angeles, CA

Study Staff

Maria Hewitt, Study Director
Mary Joy Ballantyne, Research Assistant
Timothy Brennan, Research Assistant
Gelsey Lynn, Research Assistant

Eric Trabert, Research Associate
Jill Shuman, Editor

NCPB Staff

Roger Herdman, Director, National Cancer Policy Board
Anike Johnson, Administrator
Rosa Pommier, Financial Associate

Reviewers

This report has been reviewed in draft form by individuals chosen for their diverse perspectives and technical expertise, in accordance with procedures approved by the National Research Council's Report Review Committee. The purpose of this independent review is to provide candid and critical comments that will assist the institution in making its published report as sound as possible and to ensure that the report meets institutional standards for objectivity, evidence, and responsiveness to the study charge. The review comments and draft manuscript remain confidential to protect the integrity of the deliberative process. We wish to thank the following individuals for their review of this report:

Robert J. Arceci, The Johns Hopkins University
Archie Bleyer, University of Texas
Pi-Nian Chang, University of Minnesota
Mark Chesler, University of Michigan
Maureen Henderson, University of Washington
Wendy Hobbie, The Children's Hospital of Philadelphia
John Holohan, Urban Institute
Charlie Homer, National Initiative for Child Healthcare Quality
Melissa M. Hudson, St Jude Children's Research Hospital
Ernest R. Katz, Children's Hospital Los Angeles
Nancy Keene, Author, "Childhood Cancer Survivors: A Practical Guide to Your Future"
Michael P. Link, Stanford University School of Medicine

William Long, Retired Pediatrician, Gallmann, Mississippi
Donald R. Mattison, National Institutes of Health
Ann Mertens, University of Minnesota
Jeffrey L. Platt, Mayo Clinic
Brad H. Pollock, University of Texas
Charles A. Sklar, Memorial Sloan-Kettering Cancer Center
Gilbert Smith, MAXIMUS, Inc.
G. Marie Swanson, University of Arizona
Doug Ulman, Lance Armstrong Foundation

Although the reviewers listed above have provided many constructive comments and suggestions, they were not asked to endorse the conclusions or recommendations, nor did they see the final draft of the report before its release. The review of this report was overseen by **James M. Perrin, Harvard Medical School, Massachusetts General Hospital for Children,** appointed by the Institute of Medicine, and **John C. Bailar III, The University of Chicago,** appointed by the National Research Council's Report Review Committee, who were responsible for making certain that an independent examination of this report was carried out in accordance with institutional procedures and that all review comments were carefully considered. Responsibility for the final content of this report rests entirely with the authoring committee and the institution.

Contents

List of Boxes, Figures, and Tables

BOXES

FIGURES

TABLES

CHILDHOOD CANCER
SURVIVORSHIP

IMPROVING CARE AND QUALITY OF LIFE

Summary

The treatment of childhood cancer is one of oncology's great success stories. Most children and young adults under age 20 diagnosed with cancer prior to 1970 had little hope of being cured. Since then, cure rates, as measured in five-year survival, have increased to 78 percent (Ries et al., 2002). Consequently, the size of the population of survivors of childhood cancer has grown dramatically—to 270,000 individuals of all ages as of 1997. This translates into about 1 in 640 adults ages 20 to 39 who have such a history.

Not widely recognized are the unintended consequences of this success. Along with the impressive gains in survival have come "late effects," which may impair some survivors' health and quality of life. These late effects include complications, disabilities, or adverse outcomes that are the result of the disease process, the treatment, or both. Patterns of late effects have emerged among subgroups of childhood cancer survivors that have contributed to an appreciation of cancer as a chronic disease with implications for continuing care.

As many as two-thirds of childhood cancer survivors are likely to experience at least one late effect, with perhaps one-fourth of survivors experiencing a late effect that is severe or life threatening. The most common late effects of childhood cancer are neurocognitive and psychological, cardiopulmonary, endocrine (e.g., those affecting growth and fertility), musculoskeletal, and second malignancies. The emergence of late effects depends on many factors, including age at diagnosis and treatment, exposures to chemotherapy and radiation used during treatment (doses and parts of

1

body exposed), and the severity of initial disease. Complicating the management of late effects is their variable nature. Some late effects are identified early in follow-up—during childhood or adolescent years—and resolve without consequence. Others may persist or develop in adulthood to become chronic problems or influence the progression of other diseases associated with aging. Understanding late effects is further complicated by the constant evolution of treatments. Cohorts of patients, representing different treatment eras, may experience unique sets of late effects. Some survivors of childhood cancer have positive psychosocial outcomes and there is a growing interest in better understanding resiliency among survivors.

There has been no systematic review of the policy implications of this relatively new era of childhood cancer survivorship. In this report, the National Cancer Policy Board proposes a comprehensive policy agenda that links improved health care delivery, investments in education and training, and expanded research to improve the long-term outlook for survivors of childhood cancer. In its deliberations, the Board has applied the definition of cancer survivorship used by the National Cancer Institute's (NCI) Office of Cancer Survivorship. "An individual is considered a cancer survivor from the time of diagnosis, through the balance of his or her life. Family members, friends, and caregivers are also impacted by the survivorship experience and are therefore included in this definition" (*http:// dccps.nci.nih.gov/ocs/definitions.html*, accessed March 7, 2003.). This report, focused on the experience of childhood cancer survivors following treatment, is the first of a series of reports concerning cancer survivorship. Forthcoming is a companion report on survivors of adult cancer. The distinct biology of childhood cancers, the consequences to development of children of early onset disease, and the separate care systems associated with pediatric and adult cancer contributed to the Board's decision to issue separate reports.

FINDINGS AND RECOMMENDATIONS

Developing Guidelines for Care

Recognizing the serious consequences of late effects, professional organizations and advocacy groups have recommended that an organized system of care be in place to address them. While there is general agreement that survivors of childhood cancer should be systematically followed up, there is no consensus regarding where such care should take place, who should provide it, and what its components should be.

Some aspects of follow-up care are understood to be necessary, though they may not be implemented. These include surveillance for recurrence of the original cancer or the development of a new cancer, assessing the psychosocial needs of survivors and their families, monitoring growth and maturation, counseling regarding preventive health, and testing for specific risk factors (e.g., exposure to hepatitis C following blood transfusions) or late effects (e.g., heart abnormalities, cognitive dysfunction, fertility impairment). Not well understood, however, is the optimal periodicity of follow-up contact, the value of specific screening/monitoring tests, and the effectiveness of interventions to ameliorate some late effects. Follow-up protocols are available, but they have generally been developed by individual institutions and vary in their recommendations. The lack of clarity regarding the effectiveness of interventions contributes to problems with health insurance reimbursement.

Recommendation 1: Develop evidence-based clinical practice guidelines for the care of survivors of childhood cancer.

The National Cancer Institute should convene an expert group of consumers, providers, and researchers to review available clinical practice guidelines and agree upon an evidence-based standard for current practice. For areas where bodies of evidence have not been rigorously evaluated, the Agency for Healthcare Research and Quality (AHRQ) Evidence Practice Centers (EPCs) should be charged to review the evidence. When evidence upon which to make recommendations is not available, the expert group should identify areas in need of research.

Designing Systems of Care Responsive to Survivors' Health Care Needs

In some ways, the follow-up of childhood cancer survivors is made easier by the extent to which children with cancer are treated in specialized centers of care. As many as 50 to 60 percent of children with cancer are initially treated in specialized cancer centers, but only an estimated 40 to 45 percent are receiving follow-up care in specialized clinics (Oeffinger, 2002). Institutions that are members of the National Cancer Institute-funded pediatric cooperative group, the Children's Oncology Group (COG), are required to have on-site follow-up programs, but relatively few of them appear to have comprehensive, multidisciplinary programs. The Board has developed a description of the functions of an ideal follow-up system for survivors of childhood cancer (Box S.1), but a minimum set of standards is needed to guide institutions in their development of programs to meet the wide-ranging needs of childhood cancer survivors.

According to the Board's review, four supportive care components are especially important in follow-up programs: 1) services to address the psychological implications of cancer for survivors and their families; 2) educational support through school transition programs; 3) personnel to assist

Box S.1
Functions of an Ideal Follow-Up System for Survivors of Childhood Cancer

Provide services
• Identify late effects (or the risk of late effects)
• Review prior disease history and treatments
• Conduct clinical examinations and tests
• Evaluate symptoms
• Develop plan for long-term surveillance
• Coordinate specialists involved in diagnosis and treatment of late effects (e.g, cardiologists, neurologists)
• Ameliorate late effects through rehabilitation services (e.g. physical therapy, occupational therapy)
• Provide psychosocial support
• Counsel regarding educational and occupational issues
• Counsel regarding disease prevention, health promotion
• Refer to clinical trial or other research initiative
• Provide care coordination/case management (including the transition from pediatric to adult care)
• Provide family-based care and education and outreach to survivors and their families in the community

Educate and train professionals
• Consult with primary care providers
• Consult with schools and educators
• Provide long-term perspective to oncology care providers
• Alert providers and researchers to new late effects
• Train primary care and oncology care providers

Conduct research
• Measure prevalence of late effects
• Identify etiology of late effects
• Evaluate effectiveness of interventions to ameliorate late effects
• Evaluate and modify treatment approaches to minimize late effects
• Develop standards of follow-up care

with issues related to insurance and employment problems; and 4) a plan to facilitate the transition of grown survivors of childhood cancer into adult systems of care.

A number of approaches have been proposed to address the needs of childhood cancer survivors, from follow-up clinics located in cancer centers to a national virtual consultation service organized through the internet. For many survivors and their families, geographic distance from a cancer center precludes easy access to follow-up. Most survivors are in contact with primary care providers, but the extent to which cancer-related issues are addressed in this context is not known. Few examples of collaborative practice, an approach that relies on a planned working together of oncology providers and primary care physicians, have been described. Such a model could facilitate the necessary transition from pediatric-based care to adult care as childhood cancer survivors mature into adulthood. Cancer survivors, while having some unique needs, are similar to survivors of other chronic illness. There are likely opportunities to develop efficient systems of care to address at least some of the needs of individuals with a broad range of chronic illnesses and conditions. Survivors of childhood cancer with neurocognitive impairment, for example, share medical and long-term care needs with children who have brain injuries and other neurologic conditions. Such children may be followed by a neurologist, but often do not have easy access to support services needed to accommodate adjustment to school, work, or independent living.

Recommendation 2: Define a minimum set of standards for systems of comprehensive, multidisciplinary follow-up care that link specialty and primary care providers, ensure the presence of such a system within institutions treating children with cancer, and evaluate alternate models of delivery of survivorship care.

• The National Cancer Institute should convene an expert group of consumers, providers, and health services researchers to define essential components of a follow-up system and propose alternative ways to deliver care. Consideration could be given to long-term follow-up clinics, collaborative practices between oncology and primary care physicians, and other models that might be dictated by local practices and resources, patient and family preferences, geography, and other considerations. Any system that is developed should assure linkages between specialty and primary care providers.
• A set of minimal standards for designation as a late-effects clinic should be endorsed and adopted by relevant bodies such as COG, the American Society of Pediatric Hematology/Oncology, the American Academy of Pediatrics, the American Society of Clinical Oncology, the American College of Surgeons' Commission on Cancer, and NCI in its requirements for approval for comprehensive cancer centers.
• COG members and other institutions treating children with cancer should ensure that a comprehensive, multidisciplinary system of follow-up care is in place to serve the needs of patients and their families discharged from their care.
• State comprehensive cancer control plans being developed and implemented with support from the Centers for Disease Control and Preven-

tion (CDC) should include provisions to ensure appropriate follow-up care for cancer survivors and their families.

• Grant programs of the Health Resources and Services Administration (e.g., Special Projects of Regional and National Significance [SPRANS]) should support demonstration programs to test alternate delivery systems (e.g., telemedicine, outreach programs) to ensure that the needs of different populations are met (e.g., ethnic or minority groups, rural residents, and individuals living far from specialized late-effects clinics). Needed also are evaluations to determine which models of care confer benefits in terms of preventing or ameliorating late effects and improving quality of life, and which models survivors and their families prefer.

Raising Survivors' Awareness of Late Effects

Recent research shows that the majority of cancer survivors are unaware of their risk for late effects or the need for follow-up care. They also lack specific information regarding their disease history and treatment that would be needed by a clinician to provide appropriate follow-up care. Effective interventions are available to prevent or ameliorate some late effects and a failure to receive appropriate follow-up care can be life threatening and compromise quality of life.

Recommendation 3: Improve awareness of late effects and their implications for long-term health among childhood cancer survivors and their families.

• Clinicians providing pediatric cancer care should provide survivors and their families written information regarding the specific nature of their cancer and its treatment, the risks of late effects, and a plan (and when appropriate, referrals) for follow-up. Discussion about late effects should begin with diagnosis.

• Public and private sponsors of health education (e.g., NCI, American Cancer Society) should launch informational campaigns and provide support to survivorship groups that have effective outreach programs.

Augmenting Professional Education and Training

If survivorship care is to expand and improve, additional professional education and training opportunities will be needed. Advanced practice pediatric oncology nurses have provided leadership in establishing and managing survivorship clinics, but there are relatively few such trained nurses and the oncology content in most nursing training programs is limited. Oncologists who completed their training more than a decade ago may not be familiar with the full scope of late effects now recognized, and given the cursory coverage of survivorship issues in medical texts and curricula, there is a need for continuing medical education and other educational opportunities for oncologists. Similarly, shortcomings in training of other personnel who might practice within a follow-up care system (e.g., psychologists, oncology social workers) need to be addressed. As the number of childhood cancer survivors increases, primary care providers will encounter childhood cancer survivors in their practices more often. However, these providers may miss opportunities to intervene and to ameliorate late effects because they have little experience with childhood cancer survivors and lack training.

Recommendation 4: Improve professional education and training regarding late effects and their management for both specialty and primary care providers.

• Professional societies should act to improve primary care providers' awareness through professional journals, meetings, and continuing education opportunities.
• Primary care training programs should include information about the late effects of cancer in their curricula.
• NCI should provide easy-to-find information on late effects of childhood cancer on its website (e.g., through the Physician Data Query [PDQ], which provides up-to-date information on cancer prevention, treatment, and supportive care).
• Oncology training programs should organize coursework, clinical practicum, and continuing education programs on late effects of cancer treatment for physicians, nurses, social workers, and other providers.
• Oncology professional organizations should, if they have not done so already, organize committees or subcommittees dedicated to issues related to late effects.
• Oncology Board examinations should include questions related to late effects of cancer treatment.
• Interdisciplinary professional meetings that focus on the management of late effects should be supported to raise awareness of late effects among providers who may encounter childhood cancer survivors in their practices (e.g., cardiologists, neurologists, fertility specialists, psychologists).

Strengthening Public Programs Serving Childhood Cancer Survivors

Some of the concerns of childhood cancer survivors are unique to their cancer and its treatment. However, many survivors experiencing late effects have concerns that are shared by children and young adults with other chronic illnesses and disabling conditions. Several of the key public programs that serve such children could be strengthened to assure that cancer survivors receive supportive care. These programs are housed in the U.S. Department of Health and Human Services (DHHS) and in the U.S. Department of Education (DOE). Coordination among public programs serving children and young adults is generally poor. There are differing eligibility criteria, covered services, and relationships among federal, state, and local partners. No one program has a specific mission to address the special needs of survivors of childhood cancers or to provide the full spectrum of services these children need.

An initiative aimed at improving services for children with special health care needs, if successfully implemented, could address some of these outstanding problems. The Maternal and Child Health Bureau within the Health Resources and Services Administration (HRSA) and key partners (e.g., provider and consumer groups), as part of the DHHS Healthy People 2010 initiative, have launched an effort to assure that the needs of families with children with special health care needs are met. Progress toward meeting these needs is being measured according to the following set of program objectives (Department of Health and Human Services, 2001):

1. All children with special health care needs will receive coordinated, ongoing comprehensive care within a medical home.
2. All families of children with special health care needs will have adequate private and/or public insurance to pay for the services they need.
3. All children will be screened early and continuously for special health care needs.
4. Families of children with special health care needs will partner in decision making at all levels and will be satisfied with the services they receive.
5. Community-based service systems will be organized so families can use them easily.
6. All youth with special health care needs will receive the services necessary to make transitions to all aspects of adult life, including adult health care, work, and independence.

The public programs available to help accomplish these important goals include:

1. The Maternal and Child Health Block Grant and its program for Children with Special Health Care Needs (DHHS/HRSA);
2. The Medicaid Program (DHHS/Centers for Medicare and Medicaid Services [CMS]);
3. The State Children's Health Insurance Program (S-CHIP) (DHHS/CMS);
4. The Bureau of Primary Health Care, its network of community health centers, and its supported health care professional workforce (DHHS/HRSA);
5. The Early Intervention Program (DOE);
6. Special Education Programs for Individuals with Disabilities (DOE).

All of these federal programs operate in partnership with state and local governments. Each program has its own eligibility requirements, which may be based on health-related criteria and/or income and assets.

Each state has a program for Children with Special Health Care Needs (CSHCN), funded in part through the Maternal and Child Health Block Grant. The program provides health and support services to children "who have, or are at increased risk for, chronic physical, developmental, behavioral, or emotional conditions and who also require health and related services of a type or amount beyond that required by children generally" (*http://www.mchb.hrsa.gov/*, accessed March 7, 2003). In 1989, Congress amended the Maternal and Child Health Block Grant authorization to require state CSHCN programs "to provide and to promote family-centered, community-based, coordinated care (including care coordination services…) for children with special health care needs…" and to "facilitate the development of community-based systems of services for such children and their families" (Gittler, undated). State CSHCN programs now offer training, finance community support organizations, and promote policies to further coordination of care and communication. These safety net programs have the potential to extend supportive services to survivors of childhood cancer and to provide links between highly specialized care and primary care for these children. State programs, however, currently provide an inconsistent level of services and have varying eligibility criteria that may exclude survivors of childhood cancer. States coordinate their CSHCN, Medicaid, and S-CHIP programs, but the degree and purposes of coordination differ. Medical and support services should be coordinated among federal, state and local programs.

To meet the goals of continual monitoring for special health care needs, and particularly to ensure that survivors of childhood cancer have a medical home, much stronger systems of care are needed. Community-based primary care providers and cancer center-based specialists must be educated about the programs and services available to meet the needs of these individuals and their families. Simpler communication systems that assure prompt information-sharing among all those caring for these children and young adults must be established and supported, and must be responsive to family concerns and preferences. Eligibility and program requirements that create gaps in services and restrict access to appropriate care and support services by survivors of childhood cancer must be changed. Capacity building that emphasizes the medical home, communication among primary care providers and specialists caring for and monitoring survivors of childhood cancer, and adequate support and educational services for these children is essential.

Recommendation 5:   The Health Resources and Services Administration's Maternal and Child Health Bureau and its partners should be fully supported in implementing the Healthy People 2010 goals for Children with Special Health Care Needs.   These efforts include a national communication strategy, efforts at capacity building, setting standards, and establishing accountability.

Improving Access to Health Care Services

Ideally, all Americans, regardless of medical history or employment status, would have health insurance coverage and access to affordable, quality medical care. Broad-based national health insurance reform is unlikely to take place in the near future.   Instead, cancer survivors' best hope for significant insurance reform rests with federal and state legislation that targets specific issues. Because federal legislation generally covers only federal programs, such as Medicare and Medicaid, many insurance reforms must be addressed at the state level. States could, for example, expand access to health insurance through increased support of state high-risk insurance pools. Such insurance pools provide coverage to individuals who have been denied private health insurance in the individual market. Roughly half of states have such programs and among those that do, the pools have had a limited impact in making insurance available and affordable to otherwise uninsurable individuals because of high premiums, deductibles, and copayments, and restricted annual and lifetime benefits (Achman and Chollet, 2001). A recent federal initiative helps states create high-risk pools to increase access to health coverage (DHHS press release, 2002). In the absence of major changes in the delivery and financing of U.S. health care, incremental reforms regarding particular benefits or improved patient protections must be considered carefully because when reforms increase the costs of insurance products, they can unintentionally increase rates of uninsurance. The IOM's Committee on the Consequences of Uninsurance will consider selected programs and proposals involving insurance-based strategies to expand health insurance coverage (*www.iom.edu*) in the sixth in a series of reports that address problems related to uninsurance.

Despite state efforts to reduce the number of uninsured children through S-CHIP, often through expansions of state Medicaid programs, many children remain uninsured. The Medicaid Program and S-CHIP insure more than one-quarter of American children, all of them living in families with low incomes. Many of the post-treatment services needed by survivors of childhood cancer with Medicaid coverage would be available through the Early and Periodic Screening, Diagnosis and Treatment (EPSDT) program. These Medicaid services are dictated by federal statute and include "diagnostic, screening, preventive, and rehabilitative services, including medical or remedial services recommended for the maximum reduction of physical or mental disability and restoration of an individual to the best possible functional level (in facility, home, or other setting)" *(http://www.healthlaw. org/pubs/19990323epsdtfact.html,* accessed March 9, 2003). In practice, several barriers to EPSDT have limited use of services, including a shortage of providers participating in the Medicaid program, beneficiaries not being informed of the program and its benefits, and issues related to cost.

Many individuals insured privately or through the Medicaid program are enrolled in fully capitated managed care arrangements. Managed care plans may control the use of specialists, especially those practicing outside of their plans' networks. Some research suggests that the services and specialists needed by children with special health care needs are not always available within plans and their networks. Contracts between insurance purchasers (e.g., employers, state Medicaid officials) and health plans should ensure an appropriate complement of services and range of providers to meet the needs of children and young adults with special health care needs. These requirements should be based on evidence of the effectiveness of services.

For individuals with inadequate insurance and financial resources, there is a patchwork of public and private programs for primary care. Full support of federally supported Community and Migrant Health Centers and other programs aimed at underserved groups enhances the nation's health care safety net.

Recommendation 6: Federal, state, and private efforts are needed to optimize childhood cancer survivors' access to appropriate resources and delivery systems through both health insurance reforms and support of safety net programs such as the Health Resources and Services Administration's Community and Migrant Health Centers.

Increasing Research on Childhood Cancer Survivorship

There is a growing recognition that only continued, systematic follow-up of large cohorts of survivors can reveal the full extent of late effects. Amelioration of these late effects will require investments in intervention research. Ultimately, clinical research to find targeted therapies that maximize survival while minimizing late effects will likely improve the outlook for future generations of childhood cancer survivors. In the meantime, research is needed to optimize the recovery of cancer survivors and to test ways of delivering appropriate clinical and supportive care services. This underrecognized area of research needs new support.

Several ongoing research activities will answer many outstanding questions about late effects among childhood cancer survivors. In particular, the Childhood Cancer Survivor Study, a large retrospective cohort study, will provide many opportunities for researchers. Relatively little multi-institutional survivorship research has taken place within the member institutions of the Children's Oncology Group, even though the majority of children with cancer receive their care in these settings. A renewed commitment to such research, along with investments in infrastructure to improve the ability to systematically identify and follow patients, would greatly improve the capacity and opportunities for survivorship research. While clinical, epidemiologic, and behavioral research in childhood survivorship has emerged to provide insights into childhood cancer survivorship, there appears to have been relatively little health services research to understand the health care experience and needs of childhood cancer survivors and their families.

The need for survivorship follow-up care is widely acknowledged and general recommendations for such care are available to clinicians, survivors, and their families. An active research program is needed to address the many outstanding questions regarding the necessary components of follow-up care in the identification, prevention, and amelioration of specific late effects. The Board outlines specific research priorities in Chapter 8 of this report.

Recommendation 7: Public and private research organizations (e.g., National Cancer Institute, National Institute of Nursing Research, American Cancer Society) should increase support for research to prevent or ameliorate the long-term consequences of childhood cancer. Priority areas of research include assessing the prevalence and etiology of late effects; testing methods that may reduce late effects during treatment; developing interventions to prevent or reduce late effects after treatment; and furthering improvements in quality of care to ameliorate the consequences of late effects on individuals and families.

- Both prospective and retrospective studies are needed to quantify the incidence and prevalence of adverse sequelae in representative cohorts of survivors. Establishing a population-based surveillance system for childhood cancer would facilitate population-based research efforts.
- Studies are needed of new treatments to reduce the occurrence of late effects among childhood cancer survivors and of interventions designed to prevent or ameliorate the consequences of late effects associated with current treatments.
- Research is needed on the long-term social, economic, and quality of life implications of cancer on survivors and their families.
- The COG should be supported in adding long-term follow-up to its clinical trials. There is an obligation to evaluate late effects of therapeutic interventions under study. Prospective clinical assessments are needed to learn about late effects.
- The Childhood Cancer Survivor Study should be fully supported and researchers encouraged to use data that have been collected. Resources are needed to assure completeness of follow-up of survivors and to conduct methodologic studies (e.g., assessment of the adequacy of sibling controls for psychosocial and health outcomes).
- Opportunities to study late effects within systems of care that have a medical record system that captures primary and specialty care should be explored (e.g., through the health maintenance organization [HMO] network, an NCI-supported research consortium of HMOs with population-based research program).
- As evidence emerges regarding late effects, research institutions should have systems in place to disseminate information to survivors who remain under their care, and to providers of follow-up care, in both specialty and primary care settings.

The Board has proposed this set of recommendations in the hopes of improving the outlook and quality of life of the estimated 270,000 Americans who have survived childhood cancer. Adoption of these recommendations would be responsive to the concerns of the 178,000 individuals estimated to be experiencing late effects of their disease and treatment as well as the many survivors who remain at risk for such effects. The Board has concluded that the oncology and larger health care community is not yet fully prepared to address the unique health and psychosocial needs of this population. Recommended improvements in health care delivery, education and training, and research could help complete the triumph of the success of childhood cancer treatment and extend the horizon of success beyond 5-year survival to a life free of disability and disease.

REFERENCES

Achman L, Chollet D. 2001. Insuring the Uninsurable: An Overview of State High-Risk Health Insurance Pools. Mathematica Policy Research, Inc. Princeton NJ (*http://www.mathematica-mpr.com/3rdlevel/uninsurablehot.htm*, accessed March 21, 2003).

Department of Health and Human Services, Health Resources and Services Administration. 2001. *Achieving Success for All Children and Youth With Special Health Care Needs: A 10-Year Action Plan to Accompany Healthy People 2010.* Washington DC: US DHHS.

Department of Health and Human Services, CMS. 2002. HHS to Help States Create High-Risk Pools to Increase Access to Health Coverage. Press release, November 26, 2002 (*www.hhs.gov/news/press/2002pres/20021126a.html*, last accessed January 31, 2003).

Gittler J. Undated. *Title V of the Social Security Act and State Programs for Children With Special Health Care Needs: Legislative History.* University of Iowa: National Maternal and Child Health Resource Center.

Oeffinger KC. Longitudinal Cancer-Related Health Care For Adult Survivors of Childhood Cancer (IOM commissioned background paper). 2002.

Ries LAG, Eisner MP, Kosary CL, Hankey BF, Miller BA, Clegg L, Edwards BK, Editors. 2002. *SEER Cancer Statistics Review, 1973-1999.* Bethesda, MD: National Cancer Institute.

1

Introduction

Most children and young adults diagnosed with cancer prior to 1970 had little hope of being cured (Smith and Ries, 2002). By 1997, cure rates, as measured in 5-year survival, had risen to 78 percent (Ries et al., 2002), largely as a result of the development of intensive multimodal treatments. Most patients who survive cancer have been exposed to combinations of two or three of the mainstays of cancer treatment: chemotherapy, radiation therapy, and surgery. Although impressive gains in survival have been achieved, late effects of treatment often impair survivors' health and quality of life. Success in treating disease has been tempered by the knowledge that the cure has often came at a price, which may not be manifest until many years after completion of therapy.

Survivors of the modern era of childhood cancer therapy are beginning to enter their fourth decade of life and significant consequences of their treatment have already been observed. Among the well-documented late effects are impairments in learning, growth and maturation, and cardiac function. As this cohort of children and young adults ages, it is likely that additional late effects will arise. And as treatments change, so too will their sequelae, so that ongoing surveillance will be needed to link childhood treatments to adult onset late effects. Models of health care delivery, surveillance, and research are beginning to take shape, but to date there has been no systematic review of the policy implications of this relatively new era of childhood cancer survivorship.

ROLE OF THE NATIONAL CANCER POLICY BOARD

The National Cancer Policy Board (the Board) was established in March 1997 at the Institute of Medicine (IOM) and National Research Council to address issues that arise in the prevention, control, diagnosis, treatment, and palliation of cancer. The 21-member board includes health care consumers, providers, and investigators in several disciplines (see membership roster). This report is part of a Board initiative to address issues of concern for cancer survivors with an emphasis on what happens following the primary treatment of cancer. The Board's 1999 report, *Ensuring Quality Cancer Care* (Institute of Medicine, 1999) recommended strategies to promote evidenced-based, comprehensive, compassionate, and coordinated care throughout the cancer care trajectory, but its focus was on primary treatment and it did not directly address issues related to the delivery of cancer care to children.

In its deliberations, the Board has applied the definition of cancer survivorship used by the National Cancer Institute's Office of Cancer Survivorship, "An individual is considered a cancer survivor from the time of diagnosis, through the balance of his or her life. Family members, friends, and caregivers are also impacted by the survivorship experience and are therefore included in this definition." (*http://dccps.nci.nih.gov/ocs/definitions.html*, accessed March 7, 2003). This report, which focuses on childhood cancer survivors and their care after primary treatment,[1] will be followed by a companion report addressing issues of relevance to survivors of adult cancer. Some policy issues are common to both groups (e.g., insurance and employment concerns); however, unique features of pediatric treatment and health care delivery systems led to the decision to publish separate reports on childhood and adult cancer survivorship. The Board report *Improving Palliative Care for Cancer* (Institute of Medicine, 2001), addressed the need for quality care at the end of life for those who die from cancer, including children. A recent IOM report, *When Children Die: Improving Palliative and End-of-Life Care for Children and Their Families*, further examines policies to improve care (Institute of Medicine, 2002). A Board report related to survivorship will be issued later in 2003 based, in part, on a two-day IOM workshop held October 28-29, 2002, "Meeting Psychosocial Needs of Women With Breast Cancer," with support from the Longaberger Company through the American Cancer Society.

Several background papers commissioned by the Board were essential to this report:[2]

---

[1]In this report, childhood refers to individuals under age 20.
[2]These papers are available at *www.IOM.edu/ncpb*.

- *Pediatric Cancer Survivors: Past History and Future Challenges,* Anna T. Meadows
- *Late Effects of Treatment for Cancer During Childhood and Adolescence,* Daniel Green
- *Neurocognitive Late Effects in Pediatric Cancer,* Raymond Mulhern
- *Quality of Life Issues and Cancer Survivorship,* Brad Zebrack and Lonnie Zeltzer
- *Research Involving Long Term Survivors of Childhood and Adolescent Cancer: Methodologic Considerations,* Leslie Robison
- *Cancer Survivorship: Issues Impacting Design and Conduct of Clinical Trials,* Sharon Murphy
- *Longitudinal Cancer-Related Health Care for Adult Survivors of Childhood Cancer,* Kevin Oeffinger
- *Cognitive Late Effects of Childhood Cancer and Treatment: Issues for Survivors,* F. Daniel Armstrong,
- *Long-term Survivor Programs: A Paradigm for the Advanced Practice Nurse,* Alice G. Ettinger

The Board heard from the following cancer survivorship specialists and representatives of federal agencies at the Board's quarterly meeting in July 2001:

- Anna T. Meadows, MD, The Children's Hospital of Philadelphia, provided an overview of childhood cancer survival;
- Daniel Green, MD, Roswell Park Cancer Institute, discussed late effects of treatment for childhood cancer;
- Raymond Mulhern, PhD, St. Jude Children's Research Hospital, described neurocognitive late effects in pediatric cancer;
- Leslie Robison, PhD, University of Minnesota Cancer Center, described epidemiologic and research issues;
- Sharon Murphy, MD, Children's Memorial Hospital, Chicago, reviewed clinical trial issues in survivorship research;
- Lonnie Zeltzer, MD, David Geffen School of Medicine at UCLA discussed psychosocial and behavioral outcomes in childhood cancer; and
- Julia Rowland, PhD, Director of the National Cancer Institute Office of Cancer Survivorship discussed federal research initiatives in childhood survivorship.

Perspectives on health care delivery were discussed at the January 2002 meeting where the Board heard from:

- Kathy Ruble, RN, and Cindy Schwartz, MD, of the Johns Hopkins Pediatric Oncology Program;

- Smita Bhatia, MD, representing the Children's Oncology Group;
- Mark Greenberg, MD, from the Pediatric Oncology Group of Ontario (POGO); and
- Merle McPherson, MD, MPH, from the Health Services and Resources Administration (HRSA), Maternal and Child Health Bureau, Division of Services for Children With Special Health Needs.

Margaret McManus of the Maternal & Child Health Policy Research Center addressed the Board at its July 2002 meeting regarding the financing and delivery of care to children with special health care needs.

Eric Trabert, a student at the University of Michigan School of Public Health, completed a review of programs providing follow-up care to cancer survivors in the summer of 2001 (see Chapter 5).

Invaluable insights of cancer survivors and their families were solicited through the internet by Nancy Keene (Keene, 2002), the co-author of *Childhood Cancer Survivors: A Practical Guide to Your Future* (Keene et al., 2000). Concerns related to cancer survivorship of consumers, health care providers, administrators, and others were also identified through a two-page inquiry placed in magazines and journals with a wide circulation (i.e., *In Touch* and *Oncology News International*, both published by PRR, Inc.).

FRAMEWORK OF THE REPORT

The purpose of this report is to 1) characterize the medical and psychosocial consequences of surviving childhood cancer; 2) identify essential elements of quality care; 3) explore some of the social and economic consequences facing cancer survivors such as under-insurance and employment discrimination; 4) assess the status of applied clinical and health services research; and 5) propose policies to improve the quality of care and quality of life for childhood cancer survivors and their families.

Chapter 2 characterizes the many types of childhood cancer, the frequency with which they occur, the likelihood that treatment will result in survival at five years, and the prevalence of cancer survivors in the general population.

Chapter 3 describes the trajectory of cancer care and provides an overview of the treatments of childhood cancer that are associated with late effects.

Chapter 4 discusses late effects of treatment and disease that can affect survivors of childhood cancer into adulthood.

Chapter 5 defines appropriate care for survivors of childhood cancer and characterizes the cancer care infrastructure, including sites and providers of care.

Chapter 6 reviews educational services appropriate for childhood cancer survivors.

Chapter 7 discusses two potential social consequences of cancer survivorship—insurance and employment discrimination.

Chapter 8 surveys ongoing clinical and health services research aimed at improving care and outlines research strategies to prevent and ameliorate the consequences of late effects of childhood cancer.

Chapter 9 summarizes key findings and presents the Board's recommendations for action by Congress, health care purchasers, health plans, health care providers, individual consumers, and health services researcher.

REFERENCES

Institute of Medicine. 1999. *Ensuring Quality Cancer Care.* Washington, DC: National Academy Press.

Institute of Medicine. 2001. *Improving Palliative Care for Cancer.* Washington, DC: National Academy Press.

Institute of Medicine. 2002. *When Children Die: Improving Palliative and End-of-Life Care for Children and Their Families.* Washington, DC: National Academy Press.

Keene N. 2002. Solicitation of concerns of cancer survivors and their family through survivorship listserv and provided to the National Cancer Policy Board.

Keene N, Hobbie W, Ruccione K. 2000. *Childhood Cancer Survivors: A Practical Guide to Your Future.* Sebastopol, CA: O'Reilly and Associates, Inc.

Ries LAG, Eisner MP, Kosary CL, Hankey BF, Miller BA, Clegg L, Edwards BK, Editors. 2002. *SEER Cancer Statistics Review, 1973-1999.* Bethesda, MD: National Cancer Institute.

Smith MA, Ries LAG. 2002. Childhood Cancer: Incidence, Survival, and Mortality. Pizzo PA, Poplack DG, Eds. In: *Principles and Practice of Pediatric Oncology.* 4th ed. Philadelphia: Lippincott Williams & Wilkins.

2

The Epidemiology of Childhood Cancer

INCIDENCE AND SURVIVAL[1]

An estimated 12,400 American children and adolescents under age 20 were diagnosed with cancer in 2000. Childhood cancer is rare, and the rate at which new cases develop among children (incidence) is 15.3 per 100,000 per year, which corresponds roughly to 1 in 6,500 children and adolescents under age 20 (Ries et al., 2002). The risk of any individual child developing cancer between birth and 20 years of age is about 1 in 300. There were an estimated 2,300 deaths in 2000 due to cancer in this age group, representing about 8 percent of all deaths (American Cancer Society, 2000). Cancer is the third leading cause of death among children age 1 to 4, and the second leading cause of death among children age 5 to 14 (Minino and Smith, 2001) (Table 2.1).

Genetic factors and certain prenatal (e.g., radiation, diethylstilbestrol [DES]) and postnatal exposures (radiation, viruses) are known to increase the risk of developing some childhood cancers, but for most cases of childhood cancer, the cause remains unknown. Childhood cancers are classified primarily by histology into 12 major categories using the International Classification of Childhood Cancers (ICCC). The distribution of childhood cancer by ICCC category for children and young adults under age 20 is shown in Figure 2.1.

---

[1]This section is adapted from ACS, Cancer Facts and Figures 2000, Special Section: Childhood Cancer, pp. 18-25, updated with SEER data to 1997 or 1999.

A brief description follows of the characteristics of these 12 categories of childhood cancer (defined as cancer occurring before age 20) including their associated pathology, epidemiology, and relative survival rates.[2],[3] Treatment of childhood cancer and late effects associated with disease and treatment are discussed in Chapters 3 and 4.

1. Leukemia   Leukemia is the most common childhood cancer, accounting for 25 percent of all cancer occurring before age 20. There are two main types of childhood leukemia—acute lymphoblastic leukemia (ALL), accounting for about three-fourths of leukemias, and acute myeloid leukemia (AML) accounting for much of the remainder of leukemia cases. ALL is a disease of the blood-forming tissues of the bone marrow and is characterized by the overproduction of immature lymphocytes (a type of white blood cell). ALL occurs at all ages, from birth to adulthood, but the peak incidence is between 2 and 6 years of age. In the United States, there is a preponderance of whites and males among children and young adults with ALL. Improvements in treatment have led to remarkable gains in survival, estimated at 79 percent at 5 years. Acute myeloid leukemia, a cancer of the myeloid lineage of white blood cells, occurs at all ages of childhood. The outcome is poorer for AML than for ALL, with a 5-year survival rate of 41 percent.

2. Central nervous system tumors (cancers) and miscellaneous intracranial and intraspinal neoplasms.   Central nervous system (CNS) tumors make up the second largest category of neoplasms in children, accounting for 17 percent of childhood cancers. More than half of all CNS malignancies in children and adolescents are a type of brain tumor known as astrocytomas (tumors that arise from star-shaped brain cells call astroctyes). Other common pediatric brain tumors include medulloblastomas (fast-growing tumors usually located in the cerebellum), brain stem gliomas, ependymomas, and optic nerve gliomas. The highest incidence rates of CNS tumors occur among infants and children through age seven. Five-year relative survival rates have improved over time to 67 percent.

3. Lymphomas and other reticuloendothelial neoplasms.   Lymphomas (cancers of the lymphatic system) and other reticuloendothelial neoplasms account for 16 percent of childhood cancers. The risks of Hodgkin's disease and non-Hodgkin's lymphoma, the major types of cancer in this cat-

---

[2]The relative survival rate represents the likelihood that a patient will not die from causes associated specifically with the given cancer before some specified time (usually 5 years) after diagnosis. It is always larger than the observed survival rate for the same group of patients.

[3]The intent of this section is to provide a brief overview. It is not intended for a technical audience.

TABLE 2.1 Number of Deaths and Death Rates for the 10 Leading
Causes of Death in Specified Age Groups, United States, 2000

Cause of Death[a]	Age 1-4 years		
	Rank[b]	Number	Rate
All causes	—	4,942	32.6
Accidents	1	1,780	11.7
Motor vehicle accidents		630	4.2
All other accidents		1,150	7.6
Congenital malformations, deformations, and chromosomal abnormalities	2	471	3.1
Malignant neoplasms	3	393	**2.6**
Assault (homicide)	4	318	2.1
Diseases of the heart	5	169	1.1
Influenza and pneumonia	6	96	0.6
Septicemia	7	91	0.6
Certain conditions originating in the perinatal period	8	84	0.6
In situ neoplasm, benign neoplasms, and neoplasms of uncertain or unknown behavior	9	56	0.4
Cerebrovascular diseases	10	45	0.3
Chronic lower respiratory diseases	—	—	—
Human immunodeficiency virus (HIV) disease	—	—	—
Intentional self-harm	—	—	—
All other causes	—	1,439	9.5

NOTE: Data are based on continuous file of records received from the states. Rates per 100,000 population in specified group. Figures are based on weighted data rounded to the nearest individual, so categories may not add to totals. Mortality data are not published on the age group 0 to 19 or 15 to 19.

Age 5-14 years			Age 15-24 years		
Rank[b]	Number	Rate	Rank[b]	Number	Rate
—	7,340	18.5	—	30,959	80.7
1	2,878	7.3	1	13,616	35.5
	1,716	4.3		10,357	27.0
	1,163	2.9		3,259	8.5
3	387	1.0	6	425	1.1
2	1,017	2.6	4	1,668	4.3
4	364	0.9	2	4,796	12.5
6	236	0.6	5	931	2.4
9	83	0.2	8	188	0.5
—-	—-	—-	—-	—-	—-
—-	—-	—-	—-	—-	—-
8	106	0.3	—-	—-	—-
10	78	0.2	7	193	0.5
7	130	0.3	9	180	0.5
—-	—-	—-	10	178	0.5
5	297	0.7	3	3,877	10.1
—-	1,764	4.4	—-	4,907	12.8

[a]Based on the Tenth Revision, International Classification of Diseases, 1992.
[b]Rank based on number of deaths.
SOURCE: Minino and Smith, 2001.

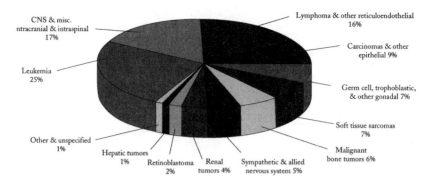

FIGURE 2.1 Distribution of childhood cancers (age 0-19), by ICCC category, 1975-1995.
SOURCES: ACS, 2000; Ries et al., 1999. Data from the Surveillance, Epidemiology, and End Results Program (SEER), Division of Cancer Control and Population Sciences, National Cancer Institute.

egory, rise throughout childhood. Non-Hodgkin's lymphoma includes T-cell lymphoma, usually found in preadolescent or adolescent males, large cell lymphoma, usually found in children over 5, and small cell lymphoma (Burkitt's or non-Burkitts's). The five-year relative survival rate has risen to 92 percent for Hodgkin's disease, and 73 percent for non-Hodgkin's lymphoma.

4. Carcinomas and other malignant epithelial neoplasms. Two malignancies in this category—thyroid cancer and melanoma—account for 9 percent of childhood cancers. Five-year survival rate is 99 percent for thyroid cancer and 92 percent for melanoma.

5. Germ cell, trophoblastic, and other gonadal neoplasms. This category accounts for 7 percent of childhood cancers. Germ cell tumors develop from testicular or ovarian cells. Sometimes these cells travel to the chest or abdomen where they may turn into a rare type of cancer called extragonadal germ cell tumor. Incidence rates and survival duration for these cancers has increased between 1975 and 1997; the 5-year survival rate now ranges between 75 and 94 percent for germ cell tumors.

6. Soft tissue sarcomas. Soft tissue sarcomas account for about 7 percent of childhood cancers. Rhabdomyosarcoma, a disease in which malignant cells arise from muscle tissue, is the most common soft tissue tumor among children under age 15. Other sarcomas are more common among those ages 15 to 19. The 5-year survival rate for soft tissue sarcomas is 71 percent, a rate that has not changed much since the 1975-1984 decade.

7. Malignant bone tumors. Malignant bone tumors account for 6 percent of childhood cancers. Peak incidence is at age 15, a trend that coincides with adolescent growth spurts. Osteosarcoma is the most common cancer in this category, which in children often occurs in the bones around the knee. Ewing's sarcoma is a rare bone cancer that usually occurs in adolescence and is more common in girls than boys. Five-year survival rates have improved substantially over time, to 65 percent for osteosarcoma and 59 percent for Ewing's sarcoma.

8. **Sympathetic and allied nervous system tumors.** Cancers in this category account for 5 percent of childhood cancers and are the most common cancers diagnosed in the first year of life. Neuroblastoma accounts for virtually all cases of cancer in this category. Neuroblastoma is a solid cancerous tumor that begins in nerve tissue in the neck, chest, abdomen, or pelvis, but usually originates in the abdomen in the tissues of the adrenal gland. By the time it is diagnosed, the cancer usually has metastasized, most commonly to the lymph nodes, liver, lungs, bones, and bone marrow. Two- thirds of children with neuroblastoma are diagnosed when they are younger than 5 years of age. Although neuroblastoma may be present at birth, it does not always proceed to become an invasive malignancy, a circumstance unique to neuroblastoma. In contrast with CNS malignancies, survival is highest among infants under 1 year of age, and declines with increasing age. Overall, the 5-year survival rate for children with sympathetic and allied nervous system tumors has improved to 66 percent.

9. **Renal tumors.** Renal tumors account for 4 percent of childhood cancers. Wilms' tumors account for more than 90 percent of malignancies of the kidney among children and adolescents, usually affecting those under age 5. Wilms' tumor may involve one or both kidneys. Between 1975 and 1997, 5-year survival rates improved for Wilm's tumor, rising from 81 percent to 91 percent

10. **Retinoblastoma.** Accounting for 2 percent of childhood cancers, retinoblastoma is a rare tumor involving the retina of the eye, or sometimes the pineal gland. Although retinoblastoma may occur at any age, it most often occurs in younger children, usually before the age of 5 years. The tumor may be in one or both eyes. Retinoblastoma is usually confined to the eye and does not spread to nearby tissue or other parts of the body. Retinoblastoma may be hereditary or nonhereditary. The hereditary form may occur in one or both eyes, and generally affects younger children. Most cases of retinoblastoma that occur in only one eye are not hereditary and are found more often in older children. When the disease occurs in both eyes, it is always hereditary. Five-year survival rate is about 94 percent and has not changed over the past two decades.

11. **Hepatic tumors.** A rare malignancy in childhood, liver tumors account for just over 1 percent of childhood cancers. More than two-thirds

of hepatic tumors in children are hepatoblastomas, most of which appear during the first 18 months of life and may be caused by an abnormal gene. The remaining cases of hepatic tumors consist mostly of hepatocellular carcinoma, which does not usually occur before age 15. Children infected with hepatitis B or C are more likely than other children to develop hepatocellular cancer. Immunization against hepatitis B may decrease the risk of hepatocellular cancer. Five-year survival rates are 54 percent for all hepatic tumors, but somewhat higher (63 percent) for hepatoblastoma.

12. Other and unspecified. Less than 1 percent of childhood cancers fall into this category.

Improvements in survival from the period 1975-1984 to 1985-1994 by type of cancer are illustrated in Figure 2.2. Survival improved from 1975 to 1994 for almost all categories of childhood cancer.

A child or adolescent diagnosed with cancer in 1994 had a 78 percent chance of surviving 5 years, while the overall 5-year relative survival rate was 56 percent for those diagnosed in 1975 (Ries et al., 2002). The largest impact on these trends has been the result of dramatic improvement in survival from leukemia, which accounts for one-quarter of cancers in individuals under age 20. The advent of newer, more effective chemotherapy treatments is the principal cause of improved survival among childhood cancer patients. Figure 2.3 shows improvements in childhood cancer survival by race from 1974 to 1998. There have been improvements in survival overall, but by 1983 a survival gap had emerged between white and blacks, which by 1998 had not closed (Figure 2.3). An analysis of overall survival, by race and treatment era, of patients treated at the St. Jude Children's Research Hospital concluded that black children with cancer fare as well as white children when treated with protocol-based therapy at a pediatric oncology research center (Pui et al., 1995). In a more recent study, however, significant racial and ethnic differences in overall survival were found among patients with ALL receiving contemporary therapy at Children's Cancer Group institutions (Bhatia et al., 2002). Relative to white patients, black and Hispanic children had poorer outcomes and Asian children had better outcomes.

The incidence rate of all childhood cancers combined increased from the early 1970s—when rates were first measured by the Surveillance, Epidemiology, and End Results (SEER) program of the National Cancer Institute—until 1991 and then leveled off and declined slightly through 1999 (Figure 2.4). Some of the increase in incidence has been attributed to improvements in diagnosis and better case identification. Mortality rates from all childhood cancers combined decreased steadily from 1975 to 1999 (Figure 2.4).

Incidence and mortality rates by race and sex are shown for the period

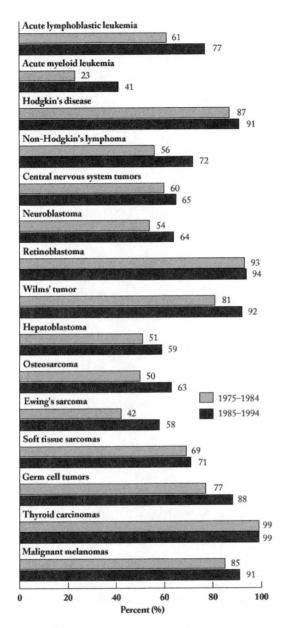

FIGURE 2.2 Five-year relative cancer survival (age 0-19), by period of diagnosis, 1975-1994.
SOURCE: ACS, 2000. Data from the Surveillance, Epidemiology, and End Results Program (SEER), Division of Cancer Control and Population Sciences, National Cancer Institute.

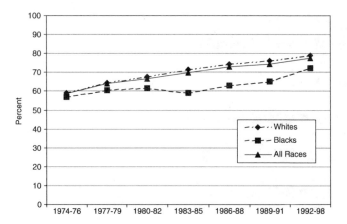

FIGURE 2.3 Five-year relative cancer survival rates (age 0-19), 1974-1998.
SOURCE: Ries et al., 2002.

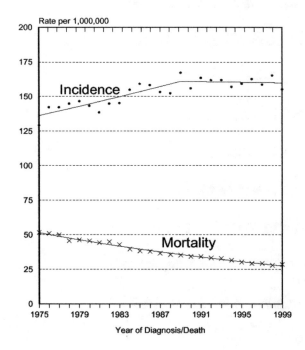

FIGURE 2.4 Age-adjusted cancer incidence and mortality rates (age 0-19), 1975-1999.
NOTE: SEER nine areas and NCHS public use data file. Rates are age-adjusted to the 2000 U.S. standard million population by 5-year age groups. Regression lines are calculated using the Joinpoint Regression Program.
SOURCE: Ries et al., 2002.

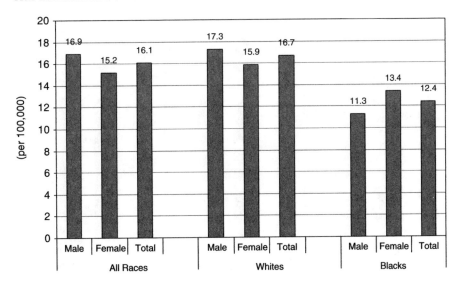

FIGURE 2.5 Age-adjusted cancer incidence rates (age 0-19), by race and sex, 1995-1999.
SOURCE: Ries et al., 2002.

1993 to 1999, the latest figures available from the NCI SEER program. Incidence rates are higher among whites than blacks (Figure 2.5) and mortality rates are higher among males than females (Figure 2.6).

Newly diagnosed cancer cases occur in roughly equal share among three age groups: younger than age 5, ages 5 to 14, and ages 15 to 19 (Figure 2.7).

Childhood cancer incidence rates are shown by diagnosis and age in Figure 2.8. Lymphocytic leukemia and CNS tumors are the predominant cancers among children under age 15. Hodgkin's disease, epithelial and other unspecified cancers, germ cell, trophoblastic, and other gonadal neoplasms are the predominant cancers among those age 15 to 19 (Figure 2.8).

THE PREVALENCE OF CHILDHOOD CANCER

The Prevalence of Cancer Among Children and Young Adults

In 1997 there were an estimated 94,800 U.S. children and young adults under age 20 who had ever been diagnosed with cancer. The prevalence of cancer among this age group was 1.24 per 1,000 (94,799/76,753,000). In other words, an estimated 1 in 810 individuals under age 20 alive in 1997 had a history of cancer (Table 2.2).

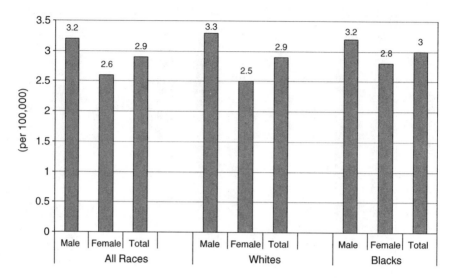

FIGURE 2.6 Age-adjusted cancer mortality rates (age 0-19), by race and sex, 1995-1999.
SOURCE: Ries et al., 2002.

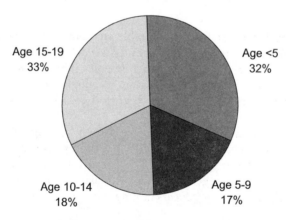

FIGURE 2.7 Age distribution of incident childhood cancers, SEER, 1975-1995.
SOURCE: Ries et al., 1999.

Estimates of prevalence for other chronic health problems among children are difficult to obtain because there are few other national disease-specific, population-based registration systems. Estimates from the 2000 National Health Interview Survey of the number of children under age 18 with selected relatively common impairments and health conditions are

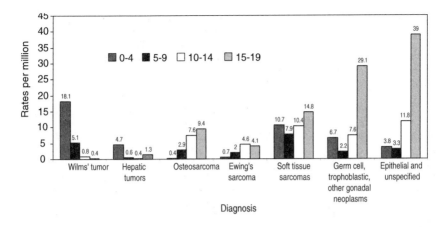

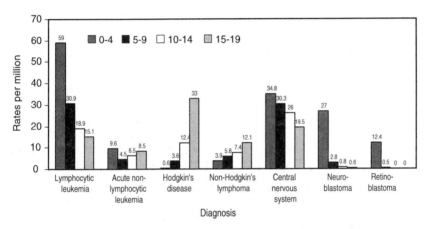

FIGURE 2.8 Childhood cancer incidence rates, by age, 1991-1995.
SOURCE: Adapted from American Cancer Society, 2000, based on data from Cancer in North America, 1991-1995, North American Association of Central Cancer Registries.

shown in Table 2.3, which helps put childhood cancer survivorship into perspective relative to other populations with special health care needs.

The Prevalence of Survivors of Childhood Cancer in the General Population

In 1997, there were an estimated 269,700 individuals of any age who had survived childhood cancer. Among the total U.S. population in 1997,

TABLE 2.2   Cancer Prevalence Estimates, by Current Age, U.S., 1997

Age	Number	Percent	Population (in 1,000s)	Prevalence (per 1,000)	Prevalence (1 per x)
All ages	8,917,906	100.0%	266,467	33.47	30
0-19	94,799	—	76,753	1.24	810
0-4	11,177	0.1%	19,193	0.58	1,717
5-9	21,026	0.2%	19,592	1.07	932
10-14	25,460	0.3%	19,046	1.34	748
15-19	37,136	0.4%	18,922	1.96	51
20-24	50,787	0.6%	17,493	2.90	34
25-29	91,716	1.0%	18,870	4.86	206
30-34	138,403	1.6%	21,020	6.58	152
35-39	216,990	2.4%	22,589	9.61	104
40-44	314,717	3.5%	21,092	14.92	67
45-49	466,974	5.2%	18,466	25.32	40
50-54	558,276	6.3%	14,542	38.39	26
55-59	667,347	7.5%	11,555	57.75	17
60-64	884,211	9.9%	10,029	88.17	11
65-69	1,192,635	13.4%	9,838	121.23	8
70-74	1,388,930	15.6%	8,771	158.35	6
75-79	1,239,461	13.9%	6,989	177.35	6
80-84	897,765	10.1%	4,620	194.34	5
85+	714,895	8.0%	3,860	185.23	5

NOTE: Cancer prevalence estimates are for January 1, 1997, from NCI's Canques program based on the Connecticut historical cancer registry (*http://srab.cancer.gov/prevalence/index.html*, accessed March 8, 2003.). The January 1, 1997, population estimate is a 2-year average of mid-Census estimates for July 1, 1996, and July 1, 1997. The 1997 population estimates will be revised in 2002 using Census 2000 data and overall prevalence estimates will likely decline somewhat because evidence suggests that population estimates made mid-Census were too low. Cancer prevalence refers to the number and distribution of individuals alive today with a current or prior diagnosis of cancer.

about 1 individual in 1,000 was a childhood cancer survivor. Among young adults age 20 to 39, the prevalence of childhood cancer survivors is 1.56 per 1,000, or an estimated 1 in 640 individuals (Table 2.4).

DIFFERENCES BETWEEN CHILDHOOD AND ADULT CANCERS

Five-year survival rates among children with cancer exceed those observed among adults (78 percent vs. 62 percent) (Ries et al., 2002). Greater success in treating childhood cancer can, in part, be explained by biological differences between adult and childhood cancers (Simone and Lyons, 1998). About 90 percent of adult cancers are carcinomas derived from epithelial

TABLE 2.3 Prevalence of Selected Impairments and Health Conditions Among Children Under Age 18, National Health Interview Survey, United States, 2000

Impairment/Health condition[a]	Population (in 1,000s)[b]	95% confidence interval
Cognitive impairments		
Learning disability [c]	4,755	4,364-5,147
Attention deficit hyperactivity disorder (ADHD/ADD)[d]	4,005	3,657-4,352
Developmental delay	2,225	1,949-2,500
Mental retardation	525	398-652
Autism	206	127-285
Sensory impairments		
Blind, trouble seeing even when wearing glasses or contact lenses	1,390	1,184-1,596
Deaf, lot of trouble hearing (without a hearing aid)	309	210-406
Conditions		
Asthma, ever	8,918	8,385-9,452
Asthma episode past 12 months	3,998	3,662-4,334
Congenital heart disease, other heart condition	953	770-1,136
Seizure past 12 months	467	360-573
Cerebral palsy	463	308-617
Sickle cell anemia	174	102-246
Functional limitations		
Limited mobility due to impairment/ health problem (expected to last year or more)	1,151	965-1,338
Need special equipment due to impairment/health problem[d]	651	513-789

[a]Categories are not mutually exclusive and should not be added.

[b]The total estimated population of children under age 18 in 2000 was 72,326,000. These estimates are based on the sample child component of the National Health Interview Survey (n = 13,376). For specific health conditions (e.g., cerebral palsy), respondents were asked if a doctor or health professional had ever told them that the child had the condition. For learning disabilities, the respondent was asked if a school representative or health professional had told them of the disability.

[c]Asked if child was age 2 to 17.

[d]Asked if child was age 3 to 17.

[d]Respondents were asked "Does . . . have any impairment or health problem that requires (him/her) to use special equipment, such as a brace, a wheelchair, or a hearing aid (excluding ordinary eyeglasses or corrective shoes)?"

SOURCE: National Center for Health Statistics, 2002, National Health Interview Survey, 2000 (machine readable data file and documentation). National Center for Health Statistics, Hyattsville, Maryland, special tabulations, NCPB staff.

TABLE 2.4 Cancer Prevalence Estimates for Survivors of Childhood Cancer (Diagnosed at Ages 0 to 19) by Current Age, U.S., 1997

Age	Number	Percent	Population (in 1,000s)	Prevalence (per 1,000)	Prevalence (1 per x)
All ages	269,679	100.0%	266,467	1.01	988
0-4	11,249	4.2%	19,193	0.59	1,706
5-9	21,279	7.9%	19,592	1.09	921
10-14	25,987	9.6%	19,046	1.36	733
15-19	38,203	14.2%	18,922	2.02	495
20-24	36,345	13.5%	17,493	2.08	481
25-29	37,937	14.1%	18,870	2.01	497
30-34	26,883	10.0%	21,020	1.28	782
35-39	23,720	8.8%	22,589	1.05	952
40-44	15,607	5.8%	21,092	0.74	1,351
45-49	15,109	5.6%	18,466	0.82	1,221
50-54	8,520	3.2%	14,542	0.59	1,707
55+	8,840	3.3%	55,661	—	—

NOTE: Cancer prevalence estimates are for January 1, 1997, from NCI's Canques program based on the Connecticut historical cancer registry (*http://srab.cancer.gov/prevalence/index.html*). The January 1, 1997, population estimate is a 2-year average of mid-Census estimates for July 1, 1996, and July 1, 1997. The 1997 population estimates will be revised in 2002 using Census 2000 data and overall prevalence estimates will likely decline somewhat because evidence suggests that population estimates made mid-Census were too low. Above age 54 estimates are unreliable because registry data are available only from 1940. Some survivors of childhood cancer could have been diagnosed before 1940 and still alive in 1997. Such individuals are not included in these estimates.

tissue.   The more common adult cancers of the prostate, breast, lung, colorectum, uterus, and ovary all arise from cells that line cavities or glands. In contrast, childhood cancers are almost entirely leukemias, lymphomas, sarcomas, and cancers of the central nervous system, primarily neoplasms that arise from non-ectodermal tissue such as bone marrow, lymph glands, bone, and muscle. This difference in microscopic type affects tumor development and response to therapy. The latency period for progression to invasive, metastatic cancer is relatively long for carcinomas, perhaps 10 to 30 years. Childhood cancers have a latency period of 1 to 10 years and many appear to derive from embryonic "accidents." Histologically, Wilms' tumor of the kidney resembles fetal kidney tissue that normally evolves into normal mature kidney tissue by birth or early infancy. Clinical experience has demonstrated that carcinomas are more resistant to radiotherapy and chemotherapy as compared with other types of cancers, especially those with embryonic features common in childhood.

The therapeutic outcomes of microscopically identical cancers in adults and children are often different. Childhood ALL has a 5-year survival rate of about 83 percent. In adults under age 65, the "same" leukemia has a much lower 5-year survival rate, from 20 to 30 percent (Ries et al., 2002). Better outcomes among children relative to adults are likely due to significant differences in the molecular, cytogenetic, and immunologic features of ALL in adults and children. For example, the Philadelphia chromosome, a cytogenetic feature associated with a very low survival, is present in 30 to 40 percent of adults, but less than 5 percent of children (Look and Kirsch, 2002).

The fact that childhood cancer occurs in the context of rapid and dramatic growth and development also distinguishes it from adult cancers.

SUMMARY AND CONCLUSIONS

Childhood cancer is rare, but with improvements in treatment there has been a dramatic growth in the population of survivors. In 1997, there were an estimated 270,000 survivors of childhood cancer; 95,000 of them were under age 20 and the balance were adults. This translates to about 1 in 810 individuals under age 20 having a history of cancer, and 1 in 640 adults ages 20 to 39 having such a history.

Childhood cancers are a diverse set of conditions, but three predominant types make up the majority of diagnosed cases: leukemia; CNS and brain tumors; and lymphomas. Five-year survival rates vary by type of childhood cancer, but overall, 78 percent of children diagnosed with cancer will be alive in 5 years. Gains in survival have occurred for most types of childhood cancer, but the greatest strides have been made in children treated for leukemia. Even though mortality rates have declined steadily since 1975, cancer remains a leading cause of death among children.

REFERENCES

American Cancer Society. 2000. *Cancer Facts and Figures, 2000*. Atlanta, GA: American Cancer Society.

Bhatia S, Sather HN, Heerema NA, Trigg ME, Gaynon PS, Robison LL. 2002. Racial and ethnic differences in survival of children with acute lymphoblastic leukemia. *Blood* 100(6):1957-64.

Look A. T., Kirsch I.R. 2002. Molecular Basis of Childhood Cancer. Pizzo PA, Poplack DG In: *Principles and Practice of Pediatric Oncology*. Fourth ed. Philadelphia: Lippincott Williams & Wilkins. Pp. 45-88.

Minino AM, Smith BL. 2001. Deaths: preliminary data for 2000. *Natl Vital Stat Rep* 49(12):1-40.

Pui CH, Boyett JM, Hancock ML, Pratt CB, Meyer WH, Crist WM. 1995. Outcome of treatment for childhood cancer in black as compared with white children. The St Jude Children's Research Hospital experience, 1962 through 1992. *JAMA* 273(8):633-7.

Ries LAG, Eisner MP, Kosary CL, Hankey BF, Miller BA, Clegg L, Edwards BK, Editors. 2002. *SEER Cancer Statistics Review, 1973-1999*. Bethesda, MD: National Cancer Institute.

Ries LAG, Smith MA, Gurney JG, Linet M, Tamra T, Young JL, Bunin GR, Editors. 1999. *Cancer Incidence and Survival Among Children and Adolescents: United States SEER Program 1975-1995*. Bethesda, MD: National Cancer Institute, SEER Program.

Simone JV, Lyons J. 1998. The evolution of cancer care for children and adults. *J Clin Oncol* 16(9):2904-5.

3

The Trajectory of
Childhood Cancer Care

In recognition of the toll its late effects have on health, cancer is increasingly being viewed as a chronic disease. This chapter first describes the entire spectrum of care for childhood cancer from diagnosis and treatment to later stages, including surveillance, rehabilitation, palliation, and end-of-life care. The chapter then provides a brief overview of the treatment of childhood cancer. Childhood cancers are a diverse set of diseases and the treatment of different types of cancer varies considerably, and within each type of cancer, the intensity and approach used may vary. For this reason, there is no clear map between a particular type of cancer and late effects. Instead, the specifics of disease and treatment dictate the likelihood of late effects. Chapter 4 explores the implications of treatment for later health and quality of life.

PHASES OF CARE

Diagnostic Evaluation

The symptoms related to childhood cancer that prompt parents to seek care are often non-specific in nature and may be similar to those of the flu or other common ailments. While symptoms may prompt parents to seek evaluation, a suspicion of cancer sometimes emerges during a routine well-child care visit. Because symptoms may mimic other common pediatric problems and because childhood cancers are rare, the correct diagnosis may be delayed. Diagnosis often begins with the primary care provider's physical examination and laboratory studies and later involve pediatric oncologists, radiologists, surgeons, and pathologists who may conduct surgical biopsies, laboratory and pathological studies, imaging tests (e.g., computed tomographic scans, magnetic resonance imaging scans), and assessments of family history.

Primary and Adjuvant Treatment

The treatment of childhood cancers is complex, involving the consideration of many factors, including characteristics of the cancer (e.g., its type, site, stage, and histology) and of the child (e.g., his or her age, presence of symptoms, and general health). In general, most children with cancer are treated using chemotherapy, surgery, radiation therapy, or a combination of two or more of these modalities. Although there are exceptions, childhood cancers tend to respond well to chemotherapy because they involve fast-growing cells, the target of most forms of chemotherapy. Many of the gains in childhood cancer survival have come through the development of combination chemotherapies (use of multiple agents) and multimodality therapy (the application of different types of treatment). While there are some accepted standard forms of therapy, an estimated 60 percent of children treated for cancer participate in clinical trials, which may involve variations in standard treatment, new combinations of agents, variations in doses of chemotherapy or radiation, use of alternate methods of administration, or entirely new approaches to therapy (e.g., immunotherapy). As information regarding late effects of treatment has emerged, therapies for childhood cancer have been informed and modified. There has, for example, been a reduction of dose or an elimination of the craniospinal radiation used to treat children with leukemia in an effort to reduce the risk of treatment-related adverse events such as growth and cognitive deficits. Since the introduction of more aggressive chemotherapies in the 1980s, however, other late effects such as damage to the heart, kidney, and hearing have been noted.

Primary Care

Children treated for cancer generally maintain their relationship with their primary care pediatrician for preventive care, health maintenance, and acute care. Following primary treatment for cancer, children resume care with their pediatrician, family practitioner, or internist. Their primary care provider must acquire information from the cancer care team on cancer treatment exposures, possible late effects, and guidance on appropriate follow-up care.

Posttreatment Surveillance and Follow-Up Care

The follow-up phase of care is the time after completion of the initial course of therapy. Children and young adults may be monitored by their pediatric oncologist following treatment for 3 years or more, depending on the disease, age of the patient, and other factors. Follow-up by pediatric oncologists typically focuses on checking for recurrence. More extensive follow-up might be offered by the treating oncologist or take place through a referral to a comprehensive clinic. Comprehensive follow-up care includes assessment of short- and long-term complications and sequelae of cancer therapies, detection of recurrent and secondary cancers, counseling about behaviors such as smoking to prevent secondary cancers, assessment of psychosocial adjustment and quality of life, and treatment for any identified late effects. Lifelong follow-up is often necessary to identify problems following cancer treatment. Such care may be provided in the context of a special late-effects clinic or become an integral part of primary care; however, evidence suggests that follow-up care is not routinely provided (see Chapter 5).

Treatment of Recurrent Cancer

Cancer may recur in the same part of the body where it was found originally (local recurrence), or it may reappear in a more distant part of the body (metastasis). The type of treatment that is selected for a recurring cancer depends on the specific type of cancer, its size, how it behaves biologically, and what previous therapy was given. Recurrent cancers can be cured, but the likelihood of cure is usually far lower than it is for the initial treatment of cancer. If childhood cancer recurs, it usually does so in the first few years following treatment. Late effects are predictably more frequent and severe in survivors treated for relapse.

Psychosocial Assessment and Supportive Care

The diagnosis of cancer in a child constitutes a family crisis—normal daily life is disrupted, and shock, disbelief, and grief may interfere with parents' ability to cope with new information and the need to make decisions. Children may be fearful and in pain, and may react with unusual behavior and moods. Families may benefit from the services of psychologists, social workers, and oncology nurses as they attempt to cope with the diagnosis and subsequent treatment. As patients and their families complete primary treatment, sources of continued support may include community-based parent self-help organizations (e.g., Candlelighters Childhood Cancer Foundation), cancer survivor day celebrations, oncology camps,

---

Box 3.1
Complementary and Alternative Medicine

Many children with cancer use at least one form of complementary or alternative medicine (CAM) to treat their disease or cope with the side effects of conventional medicine . According to a recent population-based survey in western Washington State, where insurance companies are required by law to cover licensed alternative providers, nearly three-quarters of families of children 18 and younger being treated for cancer reported using CAM. The CAM therapies reported most often were dietary supplements, followed by alternative providers, and specifically, naturopathic doctors and massage therapists. None of the parents reported using alternative medicine instead of conventional care. Parents who were dissatisfied with their child's doctor were nine times more likely to use CAM than satisfied parents. Although parents rarely forego standard therapy in favor of CAM for their children with cancer, those that do have been prosecuted for failing to obtain standard care. Providers are advised to ask parents and children of CAM use.

Given the evident widespread use of CAM, research is needed to assess its potential risks and benefits. Some herbs have been shown to increase the risk of heart and kidney problems, while certain vitamins may reduce the effectiveness of chemotherapy. CAM should be held to the same standards of efficacy, safety, and reimbursement as traditional medicine.

---

and family retreats. Cancer survivors benefit from information about late effects, health insurance, family planning (including genetic counseling), and educational and vocational issues. Those with persistent distress and adjustment difficulties may need counseling and/or peer support (Cella and Tross, 1986; Roberts et al., 1997).

Rehabilitative Services

An array of rehabilitative services may be needed following primary treatment, including physical and occupational therapy, speech and language therapy, and supportive services available at schools.

Palliative Care

Therapy intended specifically to relieve symptoms, ease distress, provide comfort, and in other ways improve the quality of life of someone with cancer is an important part of quality cancer care, but unfortunately is often not adequately provided (Institute of Medicine, 2001). This care may be referred to as palliative care, supportive care, or comfort care, and is important at any stage of cancer care management.

End-of-Life Care

One-fourth of children newly diagnosed with cancer can expect to die of their disease within 5 years, making death and end-of-life care important issues that must be addressed. In 2000, an estimated 2,300 children and young adults died of cancer. End-of-life care is diverse and can include the management of physical or emotional symptoms and limitations of function, provision of pain relief and palliation to improve or maintain the quality of remaining life, family respite, social support, and bereavement support. Hospice care is an approach to care during the final stages of life, but hospices generally have little experience with children (Institute of Medicine, 2001).

TREATMENT OF CHILDHOOD CANCER

Treatment has changed greatly over the years, with greater reliance on combinations of modes of therapy (i.e., chemotherapy, radiation, surgery) and regimens of progressively reduced chronic toxicity (e.g., reductions in radiation dose), which are intended to minimize the likelihood of late effects. Typically, a child treated in the 1960s and 1970s would receive more radiation and chemotherapy with alkylating agents than a child treated in the late 1990s. Neurologic and reproductive late effects, growth retardation, and second cancers were associated with these treatment regimens. This older cohort of survivors, now approaching middle age, is at greater risk of late effects of treatment than those treated more recently. New types of chemotherapy introduced in the 1980s (e.g., daunomycin, doxorubicin, platinum compounds, ifosfamide) are used aggressively. While they have improved survival, they have also contributed to a new constellation of late effects (e.g., damage to the heart, kidney, and hearing).

Most children with cancer are exposed to a combination of two or three therapies. According to evidence from a large cohort of 5-year survivors of childhood cancer diagnosed between 1970 and 1986 (the Childhood Cancer Survivor Study [CCSS]), 44 percent had been treated by a combination of chemotherapy, radiation, and surgery (Table 3.1) (Robison et al., 2002). The treatment of many cancers involves a unique set of therapies that can lead to a signature constellation of late effects.

Many chemotherapeutic agents are used in the treatment of childhood cancer. Table 3.2 shows the agents most frequently used to treat a cohort of 5-year cancer survivors diagnosed between 1970 and 1986 and followed up as part of the Childhood Cancer Survivor Study (Robison et al., 2002). At that time, the most commonly administered chemotherapeutic agents were dactinomycin, cyclophosphamide, doxorubicin, L-asparaginase, 6-mercaptopurine, methotrexate, prednisone, and vincristine.

TABLE 3.1 Treatment Experience of the Childhood
Cancer Survivor Study Cohort (n = 20,276)

Treatment modality	Percent
• Any chemotherapy	79
• Any radiation	68
• Any surgery	83
One therapy only	
• Chemotherapy only	6
• Surgery only	8
• Radiation only	<1
Two therapies	
• Chemotherapy + surgery	18
• Chemotherapy + radiation	11
• Radiation + surgery	13
Three therapies	
• Chemotherapy + radiation + surgery	44

SOURCE: Robison et al., 2002.

What follows is a brief and simplified overview of common approaches to cancer treatment, many of which have implications for subsequent late effects.[1]   Information on the epidemiology of childhood cancer can be found in Chapter 2.

Leukemias

Primary treatment for acute lymphoblastic leukemia (ALL) involves combination chemotherapy. However, no single standard regimen exists, as proper treatment is based on the patient's prognosis, which is determined by cytogenetic, immunologic, and molecular information. There are generally four phases of treatment:

1. Remission induction therapy uses chemotherapy to eliminate as many of the leukemia cells as possible to cause the cancer to go into remission.
2. Central nervous system (CNS) prophylaxis involves intrathecal (che-

---

[1]For more information about treatment of childhood cancers see the National Cancer Insitute's PDQ® Cancer Information Summaries at *http://www.cancer.gov/cancerinfo/pdq/treatment/*.

motherapy injected into the spinal canal) and/or high-dose systemic chemo-therapy to eliminate leukemia cells present in the brain and spinal fluid, even if no cancer has been detected there by routine testing. For this purpose, radiation therapy to the brain may be added to chemotherapy in special circumstances. Radiation to the brain is generally not used for children under age 2.

3. The third phase of treatment, consolidation or intensification therapy, begins once a child goes into remission and there are no more signs of leukemia. Consolidation therapy involves high-dose chemotherapy in an attempt to eliminate any remaining leukemia cells.

4. Maintenance therapy uses chemotherapy for two or more years to attempt to continue destruction of residual leukemia and to effect a cure.

Bone marrow transplantation is used for children with ALL under special poor-risk situations, when conventional treatment fails or as part of clinical trials.

The primary treatment for acute myeloid leukemia (AML) is chemo-therapy, sometimes followed by bone marrow transplantation. Radio-therapy is an important component for the most successful marrow trans-plant regimens for this disease. Biological therapy (e.g., immunotherapy) is being evaluated in clinical trials. Treatment for AML usually involves induction and consolidation as described above, sometimes followed by an intensification phase (another course of chemotherapy). Therapy may also involve CNS prophylaxis and radiation to the brain.

Central Nervous System and
Miscellaneous Intracranial and Intraspinal Neoplasms

Treatment for brain tumors usually consists of a combination of sur-gery, radiation, and chemotherapy. In some cases, bone marrow transplan-tation and peripheral blood stem cell transplants are also used. The specific location of the tumor in the brain, e.g., whether there is involvement of vital centers, usually determines how extensive or life-threatening the treatment is. Determinants of therapy include the tumor's classification (origin of the tumor cells), grade (degree of malignancy), and stage (extent of tumor spread). Nearly complete removal of the tumor is often possible with surgery, but complete removal of all gross and microscopic cancer is rare. Radiation therapy and/or chemotherapy usually follow surgery if the tumor cannot be completely removed. Clinical trials are evaluating radiation therapy given in several small doses per day (hyperfractionated radiation therapy). Other trials are testing ways to decrease or delay radiation therapy, especially for younger children. Researchers are also studying whether chemotherapy can be used as a means of delaying, modifying or

TABLE 3.2 Chemotherapeutic Agent Use (percent) Among CCSS Participants, by Diagnosis

Agent	Total (n = 12,455)	Leukemia (n = 4,215)	CNS (n = 1,642)
Bleomycin	6	<1	<1
Carmustine (BCNU)	4	5	3
Cisplatin	6	<1	10
Cyclophosphamide-PO	8	10	1
Cyclophosphamide-IV	40	48	7
Cytarabine-IV/IM	18	43	6
Cytarabine-IT	14	36	<1
Cytarabine-SQ	4	11	0
Dacarbazine (DTIC)	5	<1	2
Dactinomycin	20	2	2
Daunorubicin	13	33	<1
Dexamethasone	8	14	8
Doxorubicin	32	31	1
Etoposide (VP16)-IV	7	12	3
Hydroxyurea	4	4	8
Ifosfamide	1	1	1
L-Asparaginase	31	85	<1
Lomustine (CCNU)	4	<1	17
Mechlorethamine (N Mustard)	6	<1	3
Mercaptopurine (6-MP)	31	86	<1
Methotrexate-PO	28	72	1
Methotrexate-IV	22	40	1
Methotrexate-IM	4	10	0
Methotrexate-IT	36	89	2
Prednisone	47	93	10
Procarbazine	10	<1	14
Teniposide (VM-26)	5	11	1
Thioguanine	9	22	2
Vinblastine	5	1	<1
Vincristine	72	96	23

NOTE: PO = per os (by mouth); IV = intravenous; IM = intramuscular; IT = intrathecal; SQ = subcutaneous. Limited to participants with complete abstraction of medical records.

eliminating the need for radiation therapy in younger patients, as well as prior to or during radiation therapy.

Lymphomas and Other Reticuloendothelial Neoplasms

The main treatment for non-Hodgkin's lymphoma is chemotherapy (systemic and intrathecal). Radiation therapy is rarely used for the primary

HD (n = 1,685)	NHL (n = 908)	Kidney (n = 1,068)	Neuroblastoma (n = 823)	Soft tissue sarcoma (n = 1,079)	Bone cancer (n = 1,035)
22	6	<1	<1	4	25
3	20	0	<1	1	2
1	2	2	13	10	27
1	5	<1	27	17	10
22	84	8	43	56	64
2	31	<1	2	1	1
<1	22	<1	<1	4	<1
<1	7	0	0	0	0
16	<1	<1	20	8	4
<1	3	98	2	71	52
0	29	<1	<1	<1	<1
3	8	1	2	4	9
25	32	42	27	44	82
3	5	3	2	7	6
<1	20	0	1	<1	<1
<1	1	2	1	4	6
0	32	0	0	0	0
10	4	0	<1	<1	<1
39	2	<1	4	1	1
<1	29	0	0	<1	0
<1	41	0	0	<1	1
1	42	0	1	6	51
0	4	0	0	<1	<1
<1	75	<1	1	4	1
51	87	1	2	2	2
62	2	0	1	<1	<1
<1	5	<1	10	1	<1
<1	25	<1	0	0	0
30	3	1	1	1	1
55	90	91	37	73	65

Only commonly used agents are listed (greater than 5 percent use in any diagnostic group).
SOURCE: Adapted from Robison et al., 2002.

treatment of non-Hodgkin's lymphoma. The most common treatments for Hodgkin's disease are radiation therapy and/or chemotherapy, but treatment may depend on the stage of the cancer and whether the child has reached full growth. Lymphomas can start in almost any part of the body and the cancer can spread to almost any organ or tissue in the body, including the liver, bone marrow, and the spleen. Treatment depends on the stage of the disease, its location, histology, and whether symptoms are present. Bone marrow transplantation is rarely used as a primary therapy for lymphoma, but is being tested in clinical trials for certain patients.

Carcinomas and Other Malignant Epithelial Neoplasms

Treatment of thyroid cancer may involve surgery (e.g., a partial or complete removal of the thyroid), radiation therapy, hormone therapy, and/or chemotherapy. Surgery is the primary treatment of all stages of melanoma, but treatment may also involve chemotherapy, radiation therapy, or biological therapy.

Germ Cell, Trophoblastic, and Other Gonadal Neoplasms

The standard approach for childhood germ cell tumors is complete surgical excision of the tumor combined with chemotherapy.

Soft Tissue Sarcomas

Treatment of rhabdomyosarcoma, the most common soft tissue tumor among children under age 15, depends on tumor size, location, and how far and where the cancer has spread. All children with rhabdomyosarcoma are treated with chemotherapy. Surgery is a common treatment for rhabdomyosarcoma, sometimes in combination with chemotherapy and radiation therapy.

Malignant Bone Tumors

Surgery is a common treatment for osteosarcoma. Sometimes all or part of an arm or leg may be amputated to maximize the likelihood that all of the cancer is eliminated. In some patients with osteosarcoma that has not spread beyond the bone, limb-sparing surgery can be performed without a recurrence of the cancer. The cancer can be excised without amputation, and artificial devices or bones from other places in the body can be used to replace the bone that was removed. Chemotherapy is usually administered before and/or following surgery (adjuvant chemotherapy). Ewing's sarcoma, another common tumor of childhood, may be treated by a combination of surgery, chemotherapy, and radiation. Another treatment option is myeloablative therapy with stem cell support. Myeloablative therapy is a very intense regimen of chemotherapy that intentionally destroys most of the bone marrow cells, which are then restored by an infusion of the patient's own stem cells, or cells from a donor.

Sympathetic and Allied Nervous System Tumors

Treatment options for neuroblastoma are related to age at diagnosis, tumor location, stage of disease, regional lymph node involvement, and tumor biology. Four types of treatment are used, often in combination—surgery, radiation therapy, chemotherapy, and bone marrow transplantation.

Renal Tumors

Choice of treatment for Wilms' tumor depends on the tumor's size, stage, histology and the child's age and general health. The treatment of Wilms' tumor usually involves surgery to remove the cancer followed by chemotherapy. Other regimens may also include radiotherapy.

Retinoblastoma

Therapeutic approaches to retinoblastoma depend on the extent of the disease within the eye, whether the disease is in one or both eyes, and whether the disease has spread beyond the eye. Treatment options include enucleation (surgery to remove the eye); radiation therapy; cryotherapy (the use of extreme cold to destroy cancer cells); photocoagulation (the use of laser light to destroy blood vessels that supply nutrients to the tumor); thermotherapy (the use of heat to destroy cancer cells); and chemotherapy. Pediatric oncologists have modified treatment to improve survival, to preserve vision and cosmetic appearance, and to reduce second cancers. Chemotherapy is used to shrink tumors so that they can be treated focally, thereby avoiding enucleation or radiation in at least 50 percent of eyes (Friedman et al., 2000). Children who have hereditary retinoblastoma may also be at risk of developing a tumor in the brain while they are being treated for the eye tumor. This is called trilateral retinoblastoma, and patients should be periodically monitored for the possible development of this rare condition during and after treatment.

Hepatic Tumors

Surgery, chemotherapy, radiation therapy, and liver transplantation are all used to treat childhood liver cancers. Surgery may be used to take out the cancer and surrounding tissue. Chemotherapy may be administered before surgery to help reduce the size of the liver cancer and it may be administered after surgery to eliminate any remaining cancer cells. Systemic or direct infusion chemotherapy (drugs injected directly into the blood vessels that go into the liver) may also be administered. Sometimes a treatment called chemo-embolization is used to treat childhood liver cancer. This involves injecting chemotherapy drugs into the main artery of the liver with substances that slow or stop tumor growth.

SUMMARY AND CONCLUSIONS

The trajectory of care for children with cancer spans diagnosis and treatment to later stages, including surveillance, rehabilitation, palliation, and end-of-life care. This report focuses on what happens after treatment, and in particular on the care related to late effects of cancer and its treatment. Childhood cancers are a diverse set of diseases and the treatment of each type of cancer varies considerably; and within each type of cancer, the intensity and approach used may vary depending on the child's age, general health, and characteristics of the cancer. Because late effects arise following an interaction between the individual with cancer, the cancer, and the specifics of treatment, there is no clear map between a particular type of cancer or a specific treatment and an expected spectrum of late effects. Each factor must be considered in anticipating outcomes. Understanding late effects is further complicated by the constant evolution of treatments; they are, in effect, a moving target. While these aspects pose challenges to researchers and clinicians, patterns of late effects have emerged and their recognition has contributed to an appreciation of cancer as a chronic disease.

REFERENCES

Cella DF, Tross S. 1986. Psychological adjustment to survival from Hodgkin's disease. *J Consult Clin Psychol* 54(5):616-22.

Friedman DL, Himelstein B, Shields CL, Shields JA, Needle M, Miller D, Bunin GR, Meadows AT. 2000. Chemoreduction and local ophthalmic therapy for intraocular retinoblastoma. *J Clin Oncol* 18(1):12-7.

Institute of Medicine. 2001. *Improving Palliative Care for Cancer*. Washington, DC: National Academy Press.

Kemper KJ, Wornham WL. 2002. Complementary and Alternative Therapies in Pediatric Oncology. Pizzo PA, Poplack DG (eds). *Principles and Practice of Pediatric Oncology*. 4th ed. Philadelphia: Lippincott Williams and Wilkins. Pp. 1529-1540.

Neuhouser ML, Patterson RE, Schwartz SM, Hedderson MM, Bowen DJ, Standish LJ. 2001. Use of alternative medicine by children with cancer in Washington State. *Prev Med* 33(5):347-54.

Roberts CS, Severinsen C, Carraway C, Clark D, Freeman M, Daniel P. 1997. Life changes and problems experienced by young adults with cancer. *Journal of Psychosocial Oncology* 15(1):15-25.

Robison LL, Mertens AC, Boice JD, Breslow NE, Donaldson SS, Green DM, Li FP, Meadows AT, Mulvihill JJ, Neglia JP, Nesbit ME, Packer RJ, Potter JD, Sklar CA, Smith MA, Stovall M, Strong LC, Yasui Y, Zeltzer LK. 2002. Study design and cohort characteristics of the Childhood Cancer Survivor Study: a multi-institutional collaborative project. *Med Pediatr Oncol* 38(4):229-39.

4

Late Effects of Childhood Cancer

Childhood cancer survivors, though being "cured" of cancer, often experience late effects, both physical and psychological, secondary to their cancer or its treatment. Complications, disabilities, or adverse outcomes that are the result of the disease process, the treatment, or both, are generally referred to as "late effects." Late effects may be easy to identify because of their visibility (e.g., amputation) or direct effects on function (e.g., severe cognitive impairment). Other late effects, however, can be subtle and apparent only to the trained observer (e.g., scoliosis or curvature of the spine) or not directly observable and identified only through screening or imaging tests (hypothyroidism, infertility). In addition to concerns about a recurrence of the cancer for which they were treated, cancer survivors are also at increased risk of developing a second type of cancer because of either their treatment for cancer (e.g., radiation), their genetic or other susceptibility, or some interaction between treatment and genetic susceptibility.

Some late effects of therapy are identified early in follow-up—during the childhood or adolescent years—and resolve without consequence. Others may persist, become chronic problems, and influence the progression of other diseases associated with aging. For example, renal dysfunction secondary to treatment with the chemotherapeutic agent ifosfamide may be accelerated if the survivor develops hypertension or diabetes mellitus, two common adult health problems (Prasad et al., 1996; Skinner et al., 2000).

Chemotherapy, radiation therapy, and surgery may all cause late effects involving any organ or system of the body. Effects of surgery with

49

implications for survivorship may include amputation, eye removal, disfigurement, or growth abnormalities. Exposure to therapeutic agents during the rapid and dramatic physiologic and psychologic changes occurring from infancy to early adulthood can result in specific tissue or organ damage, or alteration of normal patterns of growth and development. Long-term sequelae of chemotherapy and radiation are common, may be mild or severe, and may be asymptomatic for extended periods. As many as two-thirds of survivors will experience a late effect of chemotherapy or radiation, defined as any chronic or late occurring outcome—physical or psychosocial—that persists or develops beyond five years from the diagnosis of the cancer (Garre et al., 1994; Oeffinger et al., 2000; Stevens et al., 1998; Vonderweid et al., 1996). These late effects include cognitive impairment, fertility problems, alterations in growth and development, organ system damage, chronic hepatitis, and second malignant neoplasms (DeLaat and Lampkin, 1992; Donaldson, 1993; Dreyer et al., 2002; Friedman and Meadows, 2002; Marina, 1997; Meister and Meadows, 1993; Neglia and Nesbit, 1993; Schwartz, 1995). Survivors frequently have more than one late effect, with perhaps as many as a quarter of survivors experiencing one that is severe or life-threatening (Garre et al., 1994; Oeffinger et al., 2000; Stevens et al., 1998).

The seriousness of the consequences of late effects is evident in studies of premature death following cancer treatment. In one study of late mortality among 20,227 5-year survivors of childhood cancer diagnosed with cancer from 1970 to 1986, there was a 10.8-fold excess in overall mortality (Mertens et al., 2001). Ten percent of these individuals had died by 1996. Figure 4.1 shows all-cause mortality in this cohort as compared to age-adjusted expected survival rates for the U.S. population. Survival is shown by original cancer diagnosis in Figures 4.2a and 4.2b.

Among those for whom cause of death was ascertained, relapse of the primary cancer accounted for 67.4 percent of deaths and treatment-related consequences accounted for 21.3 percent of deaths. The remaining 11.3 percent of deaths were caused by non-treatment external causes (e.g., motor vehicle accidents) or medical conditions (e.g., HIV, pneumonia) (Table 4.1). The three most common treatment-related causes of death observed were (1) the development of a secondary or subsequent cancer, (2) cardiac toxicity, and (3) pulmonary complications.

Among the Childhood Cancer Survivor Study (CCSS) cohort, the overall all-cause absolute excess risk was 8.8 deaths per 1,000 person-years. Within treatment-related cause-specific categories (i.e., excluding recurrences and non-treatment-related deaths), the absolute excess risk was 1.26, 0.27, and 0.015 deaths per 1,000 person-years for secondary and subsequent cancers, cardiac causes, and pulmonary causes, respectively. These treatment-related deaths account for 18 percent of the excess risk of death

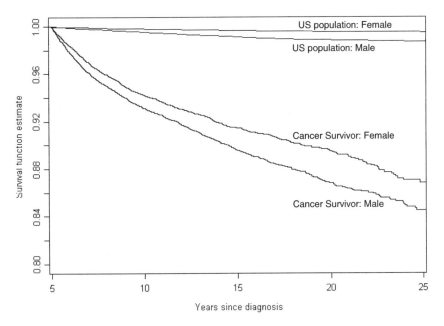

FIGURE 4.1 All-cause mortality, by sex (Childhood Cancer Survivor Study). US population: Age-adjusted expected survival rates. Cancer survivor: All-cause mortality experience from five years after inital canccer diagnosis.
SOURCE: Mertens et al., 2001. Reprinted with permission of the American Society of Clinical Oncology.

observed in this cohort. The risk was highest among females, those diagnosed with cancer before the age of 5, and those with an initial diagnosis of leukemia or central nervous system (CNS) tumor (Mertens et al., 2001; Moller et al., 2001).

The cumulative cause-specific mortality was highest for cancer recurrence (7 percent at 25 years from diagnosis) (Figure 4.2). Death rates due to subsequent cancers and other causes increased more rapidly in the time period 15 to 25 years after diagnosis than from 5 to 15 years after diagnosis.

Despite the relatively high prevalence of late effects, recent evidence suggests that survivors of childhood cancer view themselves as being in relatively good health. Only 11 percent of 9,434 members of the CCSS cohort reported that they were in fair or poor general health when recently surveyed (Kevin Oeffinger, personal communication to Maria Hewitt, August 16, 2002). This assessment may not necessarily indicate a lack of limitations or disability. People with serious chronic illness, recurring disease, or disability sometimes report being in good health because they

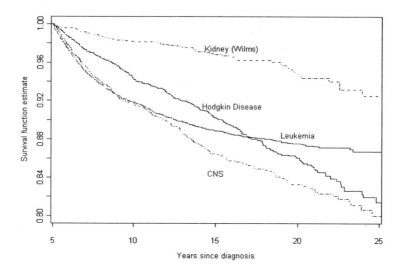

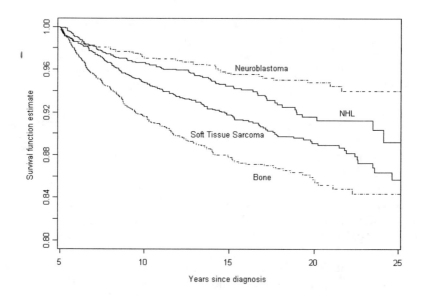

FIGURE 4.2 Mortality, by cancer type (Childhood Cancer Survivor Study).
NOTE: CNS = central nervous system; NHL = non-Hodgkin's lymphoma.
SOURCE: Mertens et al., 2001. Reprinted with permission of the American Society
of Clinical Oncology.

TABLE 4.1 Causes of Death in the Childhood Cancer Survivor Study Cohort

Cause of death	Number of deaths	Percent of deaths
Total	1,848	100.0
Recurrence	1,246	67.4
Treatment-related consequences	394	21.3
Subsequent neoplasm	235	12.7
Cardiac	83	4.5
Pulmonary	33	1.8
Other sequelae	43	2.3
Non-treatment related	208	11.3
External causes	94	5.1
Medical conditions	114	6.2

SOURCE: Adapted from Mertens et al., 2001.

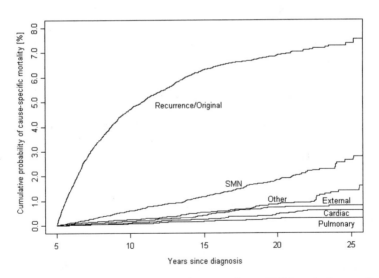

FIGURE 4.3 Cumulative cause-specific mortality (Childhood Cancer Survivor Study).
NOTE: SMN = second malignant neoplasm.
SOURCE: Mertens et al., 2001. Reprinted with permission of the American Society of Clinical Oncology.

experience benefits from their illness, for example, becoming closer to family, discovery of self and life priorities, and renewed spirituality (Justice, 1999; Kornblith et al., 1998). Researchers examined several health-related domains—general health, mental health, functional impairment, activity limitations, and pain or anxiety as a result of the cancer or its treatment—and found that 45 percent of the cohort members reported moderate to severe adverse outcomes in at least one of the domains (Kevin Oeffinger, personal communication to Maria Hewitt, August 16, 2002).

Table 4.2 summarizes some of the late effects associated with the more common childhood cancers. The next section describes how specific treatments can contribute to physical and psychosocial damage. Chapter 5 describes approaches to monitor late effects.

The most common late effects of childhood cancer include those that are neurocognitive and psychological, cardiopulmonary, endocrine (e.g., those affecting growth and fertility), musculoskeletal, and those related to second malignancies. The emergence of late effects depends on many factors, including age, exposures to chemotherapy and radiation during treatment (doses and parts of body exposed), and the severity of disease. The following section briefly reviews some of the late effects that occur following primary treatment. For a more complete discussion, see the background papers prepared for the Board (*www.iom.edu/ncpb*) and refer to comprehensive reviews that are available for both consumers (Keene et al., 2000; http://www.candlelighters.org) and providers (Dreyer et al., 2002; Friedman and Meadows, 2002; Schwartz, 1995, 1999; Schwartz et al., 1994; Ward, 2000).

NEUROCOGNITIVE LATE EFFECTS

Cognitive impairment is one of the most debilitating late effects among children whose cancer (or its treatment) involved the central nervous system. Learning problems, social difficulties, behavioral adjustment problems, and long-term education and vocational difficulties may be experienced.

There are five primary groups of children that may experience CNS-related cognitive impairments:

1. Children with tumors of the CNS
2. Children with leukemia or non-Hodgkin's lymphoma who receive CNS prophylaxis involving chemotherapy and/or radiation therapy
3. Children with tumors of the face, eye, or skull that require localized, external beam radiation therapy
4. Children treated with whole body radiation and myeloablative che-

TABLE 4.2 Selected Physical Late Effects Associated with Childhood Cancer

Cancer	Potential Late Effects	
Leukemias	• Cognitive effects (e.g., learning disabilities) • Abnormal growth and maturation • Heart problems • Second cancers • Hepatitis C (effects of blood transfusion)	• Weakness, fatigue • Obesity • Osteoporosis • Avascular necrosis of bone • Dental problems
Brain cancer	• Neurologic and cognitive effects (e.g., learning disabilities) • Abnormal growth and maturation • Hearing loss	• Kidney damage • Hepatitis C • Infertility • Vision problems • Second cancers
Hodgkin's disease	• Adhesions and intestinal obstruction (if spleen removed) • Decreased resistance to infection (potential for life-threatening sepsis) • Abnormal growth and maturation • Hypothyroidism (effects of neck radiation)	• Salivary gland malfunctioning (effect of jawbone irradiation) • Lung damage • Heart problems • Infertility • Hepatitis C • Second cancers (e.g., breast cancer in females)
Non-Hodgkin's lymphoma	• Heart problems • Hepatitis C • Cognitive effects	• Infertility • Osteopenia/osteoporosis
Bone tumor	• Amputation/disfigurement • Functional, activity limitations • Damage to soft tissues and underlying bones (radiation may cause scarring, swelling, or inhibit growth)	• Hearing loss • Heart problems • Kidney damage • Second cancers • Hepatitis C • Fertility problems
Wilm's tumor	• Heart problems • Kidney damage • Damage to soft tissues and underlying bones (radiation may cause scarring, swelling, or inhibit growth)	• Second cancers • Fertility problems • Scoliosis

continued on next page

TABLE 4.2 Continued

Cancer	Potential Late Effects	
Neuroblastoma	• Heart problems • Damage to soft tissues and underlying bones (radiation may cause scarring, swelling, or inhibit growth)	• Neurocognitive effects • Hearing loss • Hepatitis C • Second cancers • Kidney damage
Soft tissue sarcoma	• Amputation/disfigurement • Functional, activity limitations • Heart problems • Damage to soft tissues and underlying bones (radiation may cause scarring, swelling, or inhibit growth)	• Second cancers • Hepatitis C • Kidney damage • Cataracts • Infertility • Neurocognitive effects

motherapy as part of a preparation regimen for allogeneic bone marrow transplantation (marrow is received from another person)

5. Children with solid tumors or leukemia who are treated during critical developmental periods and who require prolonged and repeated hospitalizations that interfere with the acquisition of normal developmental skills.

Since leukemias and lymphomas account for nearly 40 percent of childhood cancer diagnosed in the United States and tumors of the CNS account for nearly 20 percent, a total of about 50 to 60 percent of children treated for cancer will have at last some risk of neurocognitive impairment resulting from the cancer and/or its treatment. A number of factors can contribute to neurocognitive deficits: tumor characteristics (e.g., the location and extent of the tumor), surgery (e.g., bleeding or rarely, infection), radiation therapy (e.g., dose, volume, age at administration), and chemotherapy. Not all children with CNS exposure to radiation and chemotherapy will experience neurocognitive effects, and there is no certain way to predict which children will experience them. Factors associated with higher risk for cognitive impairment include younger age at the time of treatment, the intensity of treatment, the duration of time between treatment and evaluation, and the age of the child at the time he or she is evaluated. Absences from school during treatment can also contribute to impaired academic performance.

For children with CNS tumors or acute lymphocytic leukemia (ALL), the severity of cognitive impairment following radiation therapy has been associated with the dose of radiation that is administered. Higher doses of radiation (e.g., above 24 Gy) are associated with more significant impairment, and these are the doses that are most frequently used in the treatment of children with CNS tumors. Studies of survivors of childhood CNS tumors have consistently shown substantial decreases in global IQ scores in the years following treatment, with declines of 20 to 50 full-scale IQ points noted. Lower doses of radiation (e.g., 18 Gy or less) are associated with less severe cognitive impairment. These doses are most frequently used in the treatment of children with CNS leukemia or as preparatory regimens for children treated with bone marrow transplantation. The addition of certain chemotherapeutic agents administered in high doses or injected into the spinal canal (e.g., methotrexate) significantly increases the risk for cognitive impairment. Females with ALL who received intrathecal methotrexate and cranial radiation as CNS prophylaxis have been shown to have lower levels of cognitive functioning than males. Preliminary reports suggest that cognitive dysfunction may also be more common when treatment for ALL includes dexamethasone instead of prednisone as the steroid (Waber et al., 2000).

Deficits in neurocognitive function may not be apparent in the immediate period following treatment. In one study, for example, there were no differences in the results on 16 standardized memory measures between patients randomized to receive CNS prophylaxis with either 18 Gy cranial irradiation or high-dose intravenous methotrexate (Mulhern et al., 1988). Subsequent periodic evaluation of these patients, however, showed declines in scores in both treatment groups (Ochs et al., 1991).

Studies of cognitive late effects in children treated for ALL and CNS tumors suggest that nonverbal abilities are most impaired, including short-term memory, processing speed, visual-motor integration, sequencing ability, and attention and concentration. These effects are common to other types of acquired brain injury. Such impairments can affect school performance, learning, and social function. Children may have difficulty completing work in the classroom, and may spend substantially more time completing homework assignments. There may also be difficulties with handwriting, organizing material on a page, lining up columns for arithmetic problems, and accurately responding to standardized testing forms that require shading responses on a computerized record. Problems with inattention may contribute to difficulties in completing tasks or following conversations. This complex of cognitive late effects contributes to educational difficulties with reading, language development, and complex mathematics (e.g., multiplication and division). Special education services are often required to overcome recognized learning difficulties.

A large retrospective cohort study of 593 adult survivors of childhood ALL and 409 sibling controls demonstrated that ALL survivors have a greater likelihood of being placed in special education or learning disabled programs than their siblings, but that most are able to compensate and adapt to overcome these problems (Challinor and Karl, 1995; Haupt et al., 1994, 1995). On average, ALL survivors had lower grades, higher enrollment rates in special education or learning disability programs (four times greater than their siblings), and when enrolled, spent a longer time in these programs than did their siblings (Table 4.3). Cancer survivors were also at higher risk of missing school for long periods and repeating a year of school. Most ALL survivors had rates of high school graduation, college entry, and college graduation that were similar to those of their brothers and sisters, suggesting that remediation was successful. Only survivors treated with 24 Gy or more of cranial radiation and those diagnosed at a preschool age were at higher risk for poor educational performance; this group was identified by investigators as in need of targeting for remediation.

Participants in this study had to be at least 18 years old by 1990, to have been treated for ALL before age 20, to have survived at least 2 years after diagnosis, to be in remission, and to be receiving no leukemic therapy at follow-up. Nearly one-quarter (24 percent) of the sample had been diagnosed under age 6. Survivors were old enough to have finished high school and many had finished college. The educational outcomes of children currently treated on some of the intensive chemotherapy protocols in the 1990s are not yet available (D. Armstrong, University of Miami School of Medicine, personal communication to Maria Hewitt, March 28, 2002).

Some small single-institution studies have found relatively high rates of use of special education. In one study, 12 of 24 survivors of childhood ALL treated with 18 Gy of craniospinal irradiation and intrathecal chemotherapy (methotrexate) had received some type of special education service when assessed 4 to 5 years from the time of their diagnosis (Rubenstein et al., 1990). Another study conducted in The Netherlands found that 7 of 28 children treated for ALL with chemotherapy and radiation and assessed 10 years later had received special education services, a rate much higher than for their siblings (4 percent). There were no differences in special education placements between children treated with chemotherapy without radiation and their siblings. However, they had significant deficits in auditory memory and fine-motor functioning (Kingma et al., 2001). Some estimate that as many as 70 to 80 percent of high-risk children (e.g., those with CNS tumors treated with high-dose, whole-brain radiation under age 4) may need special education services (Armstrong et al., 1999; Packer et al., 1987).

As discussed above, neurocognitive deficits may not be evident in the period immediately following treatment. Studies of children with CNS tumors show that they generally do not lose abilities that had been acquired prior to treatment. Instead, the children appear to improve their skills in some areas, but at a substantially slower rate than healthy children. Other skills, which would be expected to emerge in a predictable developmental sequence in normal children, may not emerge because the underlying brain structures fail to develop. Learning disabilities are defined in terms of recognized discrepancies between intellectual functioning and academic achievement. A discrepancy may not be observed shortly following treatment, but may become evident at a later time. Because the kinds of impairments experienced by children with cancer emerge over time, neurocognitive evaluations need to be conducted on a schedule that anticipates areas of deficit (Iuvone et al., 2002). Assessment tools used in these evaluations should focus on the specific areas of potential deficits that are associated with the type of brain injury resulting from cancer treatment. This may require neuropsychological testing that is typically not provided by the educational system and the use of tests that fall outside the scope of those routinely used in educational planning.

The evidence regarding neurocognitive deficits associated with cancer treatment is being used to moderate treatments to reduce these effects. The results of ongoing studies to maintain and improve survival while minimizing cognitive impairment, however, will not be available for another 5 to 10 years. Preliminary results of assessments of interventions to remediate treatment-related cognitive effects using a psychologically based outpatient rehabilitation program appear promising (Butler et al., 2002). Educational programs of relevance to cancer survivors are discussed in Chapter 6.

PSYCHOSOCIAL AND BEHAVIORAL LATE EFFECTS

"The experience of completing cancer treatment has two faces—one of celebration and hope, one of uncertainty and fear" (Haase and Rostad, 1994, p. 1490). Cancer may have psychological, social, and spiritual or existential effects secondary to worry about many aspects of survivorship, including the risk of relapses, dying, more treatments, potential problems with sexuality and fertility, body image, school and work performance, and social and family relationships (Gray et al., 1992; Rait et al., 1992; Roberts et al., 1998; Weigers et al., 1998). "Quality of life" studies assess the frequency of untoward consequences of disease and factors associated with them.

Despite periods of intense stress, most survivors achieve normal levels of psychological and social functioning, and families adapt well. All survivors, however, even those apparently doing quite well, experience at least occasional problems in social adjustment and continue to be concerned about their medical and social futures. There is a small but significant minority of survivors who remain seriously troubled and are impaired by their psychological problems. The size of this group, and the nature and extent of their problems are not fully known (Fritz et al., 1988; Gray et al., 1992; Greenberg et al., 1989; Hobbie et al., 2000; Kazak and Meadows, 1989; Koocher and O'Malley, 1981; Kupst et al., 1995; Moore et al., 1987;

TABLE 4.3 Enrollment in Special Education Programs Among Survivors of Childhood Acute Lymphoblastic Leukemia Relative to Sibling Controls, by Time from Diagnosis[a]

Educational Outcome	Before diagnosis Event rate[b]	RR[c]	After diagnosis Event rate[b]	RR[c]
Special education				
Total	3.8	1.4	9.5	3.4*
Age at diagnosis, y				
0-5			12.3	4.5*
≥6			7.7	2.8*
Cranial radiation, Gy				
None			5.8	2.1
18			7.2	2.6*
24			11.4	4.1*
Intrathecal methotrexate, mg				
None			11.5	4.1*
<83			11.2	4.1*
≥83			5.5	2.0*
Learning disabled				
Total	5.1	1.4	13.3	3.6*
Age at diagnosis, y				
0-5			17.5	4.7*
≥6			10.8	2.9*
Cranial radiation, Gy				
None			6.0	1.6
18			5.4	1.4
24			19.6	5.3*
Intrathecal methotrexate, mg				
None			12.5	3.3*
<83			18.2	4.9*
≥83			6.9	1.9
Gifted and talented				
Total	7.0	1.0	7.0	1.0
Age at diagnosis, y				
0-5			4.2	0.6
≥6			8.9	1.2
Cranial radiation, Gy				
None			5.7	0.8
18			8.5	1.2
24			6.2	0.9
Intrathecal methotrexate, mg				
None			8.0	1.1
<83			5.2	0.7
≥83			9.1	1.3

[a]Only survivors diagnosed before 18 years of age were considered.
[b]Events per 1,000 person-years.

From diagnosis through 2 y after diagnosis		After 3 y from diagnosis	
Event rate[b]	RR[c]	Event rate[b]	RR[c]
5.5	2.0	11.3	4.1*
8.1	2.9	13.0	4.7*
4.9	1.8	9.7	3.5*
0	—	8.8	3.2
1.4	0.5	11.2	4.0*
10.8	3.9*	11.6	4.2*
16.2	5.9*	10.3	3.7*
4.9	1.8	13.6	4.9*
3.0	1.1	7.5	2.7*
13.2	3.5*	13.4	3.6*
24.7	6.6*	16.3	4.4*
0.9	2.9*	10.7	2.9*
0	—	9.1	2.4*
4.4	1.2	6.1	1.6
25.0	6.7*	17.8	4.8*
10.8	2.9	12.9	3.5*
21.8	5.8*	16.7	4.5*
6.1	1.6	7.6	2.0
11.3	1.6	5.1	0.7
4.1	0.6	4.2	0.6
12.8	1.8	6.0	0.8
17.5	2.4	0	—
15.2	2.1*	4.0	0.6
6.2	0.9	6.2	0.9
10.8	1.5	7.3	1.0
10.0	1.4	3.5	0.5
12.7	1.8	6.3	0.9

[c]RR indicates relative risk and compares the event rate in survivors (shown) to the event rate in controls (not shown).

*P < 0.05.

SOURCE: Haup et al., 1994 (reprinted with permission).

Mulhern et al., 1989; Stuber et al., 1996; Van Dongen-Melman and Sanders-Woudstra, 1986; Wasserman et al., 1987). A syndrome similar to postraumatic stress disorder (PTSD)[1] has been reported in adolescent and young adult survivors (Hobbie et al., 2000; Meeske et al., 2001) and in mothers, fathers, and siblings of childhood cancer survivors (Kazak et al., 199, 2002). Stress, either immediate or delayed, in response to childhood cancer is not surprising given the strenuous, invasive, and often painful nature of the treatments involved. PTSD is associated with anxiety and psychological distress, and may interfere with achievement of developmental milestones. Eiser and colleagues, however, in their systematic review of the literature on the psychological consequences of cancer found no higher prevalence of PTSD among childhood survivors in studies that included control groups (Eiser et al., 2000). More research in this area is needed to better understand the nature and extent of psychological distress among survivors of childhood cancer.

Some research has shown limitations of social functioning among children of school age. Survivors of CNS tumors, for example, have been shown to be less popular with other children (Noll et al., 1997). Studies of adult survivors of childhood cancer have shown poorer functioning in the areas of friendships and social contacts (Mackie et al., 2000). Preliminary results of a study of marriage among members of the Childhood Cancer Survivor Study suggest that adult survivors of childhood cancer marry at lower rates than expected, especially survivors of CNS tumors (Rauck et al., 1999).

Psychosocial interventions to address these concerns can include psychological, emotional, peer, or education support; social skills training; adjustment counseling; family counseling; therapeutic play; cognitive-behavioral interventions; and group or individual psychotherapy (Cohen and Walco, 1999; Kazak et al., 1999; Schwartz, 1999; Van Dongen-Melman, 2000; Walker, 1989). Applied research is needed to identify survivors and their families who are likely to benefit from services, and the relative success of interventions in improving quality of life. Also needed is research to identify the psychosocial issues and service needs of racial and ethnic minority populations and families of low socioeconomic status.

---

[1]Diagnostic criteria for posttraumatic stress disorder include 1) experiencing or witnessing an event that is perceived as a threat to life or the bodily integrity of self or loved one, with an accompanying reaction of intense fear, horror, or helplessness (in children, this may be expressed by disorganized or agitated behavior); 2) persistent re-experiencing of the event; 3) avoidance of things, events, or people that remind one of the event or numbing of responsiveness; and 4) persistent symptoms of increased arousal. The disturbance lasts for more than 1 month and causes clinically significant distress or impairment (American Psychiatric Association, 1998; Rourke et al., 1999).

Survivors with substantial physical late effects, learning problems, or relapse are more likely than survivors without late effects to show evidence of lower self-esteem, poorer adjustment, and worse quality of life (Chen et al., 1998; Fritz et al., 1988; Kazak et al., 1994; Koocher et al., 1980; Kupst and Schulman, 1988; Moore et al., 1987; Mulhern et al., 1989; Van Dongen-Melman and Sanders-Woudstra, 1986; Zebrack and Chesler, 2002; Zeltzer, 1993). Other research suggests that survivors diagnosed at an older age (Kupst et al., 1995) or who are older at the time of inquiry (Barakat et al., 1997; Elkin et al., 1997) show more negative psychosocial outlooks, as do those who are from families of lower socioeconomic status (Greenberg et al., 1997; Kupst and Schulman, 1988) or who have experienced more concurrent stress (Barakat et al., 1997). Others have identified high dose radiation, younger age at diagnosis, and female gender as risk factors for mood disturbance in long-term survivors (Zeltzer et al., 1997).

A recent report from the Childhood Cancer Survivor Study indicates that certain sociodemographic characteristics (i.e., female gender, lower household income, lower educational attainment, not being employed) are associated with an increased risk for depression and somatic distress among both leukemia and lymphoma survivors and their sibling controls (Zebrack et al., 2002). These sociodemographic characteristics are generally recognized as risk factors for mental illness in the general population. Only exposure to intensive chemotherapy added to childhood cancer survivors' risk for reporting somatic distress. These findings from the largest cohort of childhood cancer survivors to date (over 16,000 survivors diagnosed before age 18 and ranging in age from 14 to 52 at time of study) have led the authors to theorize that psychosocial distress results from limited educational and employment opportunities that are secondary to late effects of chemotherapy and cancer-related social disruptions at critical developmental life stages (Zebrack et al., 2002). Other investigators examining outcomes among cancer survivors have suggested that increased anxiety and depression in children who have had treatment for childhood cancer may be a consequence of perceived or real academic underachievement (Brouwers et al., 2002).

There are anecdotal reports of psychological growth among survivors in response to childhood cancer (Eiser and Havermans, 1994), and in several studies childhood cancer survivors were significantly healthier in psychosocial terms or more appreciative of life than population norms or healthy controls (Arnholt et al., 1993; Cella and Tross, 1986; Elkin et al., 1997; Maggiolini et al., 2000; Weigers et al., 1998). These findings suggest a degree of resiliency and positive adaptation among some long-term survivors of childhood cancer. However, the extent to which psychological growth and meaning attributed to the cancer experience exists among survivors has yet to be determined and deserves further research.

Childhood cancer affects entire families (Chesler and Barbarin, 1987), and the health and well-being of the childhood cancer survivor is inextricably linked to the health and well-being of his or her own parents, siblings, and eventually spouses and significant others, as well as offspring. An example of the familial effect of childhood cancer is the finding that siblings of children with cancer have more somatic symptoms and poorer health care than healthy controls (Barbarin et al., 1995; Dolgin et al., 1997; Sahler et al., 1994; Sargent et al., 1995; Zeltzer et al., 1996). The long-term implications for siblings of childhood cancer survivors are unknown, and studies using these siblings as control groups may in fact lead to underestimation of problems among survivors.

Risky Behaviors

Some evidence suggests that childhood cancer survivors engage in behaviors that are likely to further increase their risk of subsequent cancer and other chronic illnesses. In one study, survivors had higher rates of alcoholism than the general population (Lansky et al., 1986). Despite their increased risks for second cancers, smoking rates among survivors were equal to those in the general U.S. population according to some studies (Emmons et al., 2002; Hollen and Hobbie, 1993; Hollen and Hobbie, 1996; Tao et al., 1998; Troyer and Holmes, 1988). Certain survivors are at particularly high risk for smoking-related health effects, especially individuals who received potentially pulmonary-damaging treatments such as bleomycin, or cardiotoxic treatments such as anthracyclines. According to a survey of 40 young adult survivors, 47 percent reported trying tobacco, 17 percent continued to smoke, and 12 percent reported binge drinking (Mulhern et al., 1995).

Survivors were less likely to quit smoking as compared with sibling controls according to one study (Haupt et al., 1992); however, another study showed no significant differences among quit rates between survivors and sibling controls (Tao et al., 1998). Survivors were significantly less likely to initiate smoking, but once having started, they were as likely as controls to become regular smokers (Tao et al., 1998). Furthermore, both survivor and sibling smokers reported substantial habits (greater than 1/2 pack per day). Childhood cancer survivors, particularly if they are male, with high rates of anxiety, depression, or self-esteem deficits, limited vocational potential, and physical health or functioning deficits may be especially likely to engage in risk-taking behaviors. In contrast, females in the general population are more likely to experience anxiety or depression, low self-esteem, and low vocational potential (Nolen-Hoeksema, 1987), which may secondarily increase their risk-taking behaviors. Treatment variables, such as exposure to cranial irradiation and demographic variables such as age at diagnosis, have been demonstrated to significantly and negatively affect educational attainment in long-term survivors of childhood leukemia (Haupt et al., 1994). Treatment intensity during childhood may serve as a risk factor for adult survivors' health-compromising behaviors as the result of neuropsychological deficits that arise from cancer treatment (Chen et al., 1998; Hollen, 2000).

It is still unclear which treatment factors (type and level of chemotherapy or radiation therapy) and quality of life issues (psychological distress, vocational potential, or physical health and functioning) will best predict high-risk behavior. Investigators have found lower risk-taking behaviors (i.e., smoking, alcohol use, illicit drug use) among resilient adolescents, those with good decision-making abilities, and those described as having an easygoing temperament, high self-esteem, and a sense of control and autonomy (Hollen et al., 1997; Hollen et al., 2001).

It is also not well understood how sociodemographic variables such as age at diagnosis, gender, ethnicity or socioeconomic status influence risk behavior. Limited investigations into the role of race and ethnicity in health behavior outcomes for childhood cancer survivors have not demonstrated ethnic differences in health behavior outcomes (Mulhern et al., 1995); yet, race/ethnicity and socioeconomic status are considered predisposing (as well as confounding) factors for increased vulnerability of young people engaging in risk-taking behaviors (Irwin, 1993). It may be that small sample size in reported survivor studies has limited the power for examining race and ethnicity as risk factors.

Some adult survivors engage in behaviors that increase their risk of disease and disability. Adult survivors of childhood cancer were less likely to smoke than the general population, but 17 percent were still current smokers according to an analysis of behaviors of 9,709 adult survivors participating in the Childhood Cancer Survivor Study (Emmons et al., 2002). Survivors who had received chest radiation or anthracyclines were no less likely to smoke than other survivors. These studies underscore the need for survivors to receive counseling regarding high-risk behaviors. Preliminary results from studies of smoking cessation interventions among childhood cancer survivors show success in helping smokers to quit (Emmons et al., 2002).

HEART AND LUNG LATE EFFECTS

Childhood cancer survivors with a history of exposure to certain chemotherapeutic agents (i.e., anthracyclines, notably daunomycin and doxorubicin) or thoracic radiotherapy are at increased risk for late-onset cardiac and pulmonary toxicity. According to recent studies of the CCSS cohort, 18 percent of survivors of childhood brain tumors reported one or more cardiovascular condition (Gurney et al., 2003). Among the entire cohort, survivors faced an increased risk of a number of pulmonary complications including lung fibrosis, recurrent pneumonia, chronic cough, use of supplemental oxygen, abnormal chest wall, exercise-induced shortness of breath, and bronchitis (Mertens et al., 2002). Chest radiation was associated with a 3.5 percent cumulative incidence of lung fibrosis at 20 years after diagnosis.

Chemotherapy-Induced Heart Damage

Anthracyclines have been used in the treatment of several childhood cancers, including Hodgkin's and non-Hodgkin's lymphomas, soft tissue sarcoma, ALL, and Wilms' tumor. Being female, young age at treatment, higher rate of administration or cumulative dose, and concurrent treatment with chest (mantle) radiation are independent risk factors that contribute to the development of heart abnormalities. The use of drugs that protect the heart (e.g., dexrazoxane) is under investigation and appears to decrease acute toxicity secondary to anthracyclines (Wexler, 1998). Further longitudinal studies will be needed to ascertain their long-term protective action.

Most survivors who develop echocardiographic evidence of left ventricular dysfunction after treatment with an anthracycline will likely remain asymptomatic, but longitudinal studies suggest that a significant proportion of those treated will experience progressive changes and may develop congestive heart failure (Grenier and Lipshultz, 1998; Lipshultz et al., 1995). Within the first 10 years after treatment, about 4 to 5 percent of survivors will have overt congestive heart failure (Lipshultz et al., 1991; Steinherz et al., 1991). However, the incidence of echocardiographically demonstrated severe left ventricular dysfunction increases with the duration of follow-up, and thus, the long-term incidence of survivors who will become symptomatic is likely considerably higher. Late cardiac failure may be induced among those with heart damage by alcohol consumption, physical inactivity, or rapid growth. Importantly, in female survivors, the initial presentation of congestive heart failure may be abruptly precipitated by pregnancy or delivery (Grenier and Lipshultz, 1998; Shan et al., 1996).

In the general population, early identification and aggressive management of left ventricular dysfunction contribute to reductions in morbidity and mortality and improved quality of life. Treatment of asymptomatic patients is associated with a delay in the onset of symptomatic disease, improvement in ejection fractions (percentage of blood ejected from the heart with each beat), and lower rates of death or hospitalization for heart failure (Exner et al., 1999). Treatment of co-morbid conditions and risk factors, such as hypertension, diabetes mellitus, dyslipidemia, and smoking, has been shown to reduce the risk for developing heart failure (McKelvie et al., 1999). Treatment of congestive heart failure with either an angiotensin-converting enzyme inhibitor or a beta-adrenergic blocking agent (standard drug therapy) results in improved quality of life and reduced mortality rates.

Based on the benefits of early identification, risk modification, and aggressive management of adults in the general population with cardiomyopathy, there is general consensus that periodic monitoring of left ventricular function of asymptomatic survivors who were treated with moderate to high doses of anthracyclines is appropriate, especially for females and those treated at a younger age or with chest radiation (Grenier and Lipshultz, 1998; Lipshultz et al., 1991).

Chemotherapy can also damage the lung (Abid et al., 2001; Ginsberg and Comis, 1982; Mertens et al., 2002; O'Driscoll et al., 1990, 1995). Bleomycin, for example, causes fibrosis of the lung that reduces lung function. Pulmonary toxicity, when it occurs, can cause significant disability. For individuals treated with bleomycin, there is a subsequent risk posed by oxygenation after anesthesia (Goldiner et al., 1978; Goldiner and Schweizer, 1979).

Radiation-Induced Heart and Lung Damage

Radiation damage to the heart has been recognized since the 1960s, and consequently, total pericardial (tissue covering the heart) radiation doses have been reduced to minimize cardiovascular effects. A cohort of patients who survived radiation treatment administered before 1974 suffered high rates of cardiovascular damage. Among 635 pediatric Hodgkin's disease patients (under age 21) treated using radiotherapy at Stanford University between 1961 and 1991, 7 of 12 deaths observed 3 to 22 years after radiation were due to acute myocardial infarction (Hancock et al., 1993; Leonard et al., 2000). Radiation-related valvular disease (Carlson et al., 1991), pericardial thickening, and ischemic heart disease have been observed among those with radiation exposure to the heart. Investigators have concluded that symptomatic disease may not appear for many years following mediastinal irradiation (Green et al., 1987). Little is known of the effects of lower dose radiation therapy currently in use (from 15 to 25 Gy).

Radiation therapy and chemotherapy (carmustine [BCNU], high dose cyclophosphamide) can also contribute to lung dysfunction and disease. Chest and thoracic irradiation can adversely affect lung function, for example, by inhibiting chest wall growth that may in turn diminish lung volume. These pulmonary effects may be subtle and may be only indirectly associated with cancer treatment. Lung volume may be reduced, for example, if individuals avoid exercise that has become difficult.

LATE EFFECTS INVOLVING ENDOCRINE FUNCTION AND FERTILITY

Endocrine complications are among the most prevalent late effects experienced by survivors of childhood cancer, affecting 20 to 50 percent of survivors who have been followed into adulthood (Friedrich, 2001; Gurney et al., 2003; Oberfield and Sklar, 2002). A common delayed effect of radiation therapy for Hodgkin's disease, brain tumors, and ALL is thyroid dysfunction, including hypothyroidism, hyperthyroidism, goiter, or nodules (Sklar et al., 2000). The high risk of thyroid disease persists more than 25 years after patients receive radiation therapy for Hodgkin's disease. The consequences of cranial irradiation can include growth hormone deficiency, delayed or precocious puberty, and hypopituitarism. Effects depend on dose, age at time of exposure, and gender. Hormonal alterations can be successfully treated, but concerns have been raised that such treatment may, in some cases, increase the risk of the development of second cancers. A recent study, for example, found an increased risk of second malignant neoplasms in childhood cancer survivors who had received growth hormone therapy for growth hormone deficiency following cranial irradiation for childhood cancer (Sklar et al., 2002). Other studies of more heterogeneous populations have not identified an increased risk of leukemia among patients treated with growth hormone, an unknown number of whom were childhood cancer survivors (Fradkin et al., 1993). Additional research is needed to clarify the risks associated with hormone therapy.

Growth

Linear growth (height) may be inhibited by cranial irradiation through its effect on the hypothalamic/pituitary axis (see also effects on the skeleton and muscles below). The effect is dose- and age-dependent. Patients treated with large doses of whole-brain radiotherapy, usually for brain tumors, are likely to have severe growth hormone deficiency necessitating hormone replacement. Lower doses of radiation, those typical for treatment of leukemia, may result in less dramatic retardation of growth. The growth of children treated for leukemia is often impaired when exposed to total body radiation and/or high-dose chemotherapy prior to bone marrow transplantation (Clement-De Boers et al., 1996; Hovi et al., 1990; Huma et al., 1995; Sanders et al., 1986; Wingard et al., 1992).

Spinal radiotherapy can compound loss in stature secondary to the direct inhibition of vertebral body growth (Donaldson et al., 1988; Probert and Parker, 1975; Riseborough et al., 1976). Early onset of puberty is common after cranial radiation, further reducing ultimate height. The younger the child is at the time of radiation, the earlier the onset of puberty.

Growth hormone treatment increases growth velocity in patients at risk for growth retardation (Giorgiani et al., 1995; Leiper et al., 1987; Papadimitriou et al., 1991). Growth hormone administration beginning shortly after completion of therapy is being assessed. Close monitoring of growth is recommended but may not be sufficient. Early onset of puberty with consequent early epiphyseal fusion will prevent successful interventions.

The sensitivity of adipose tissue to radiation may lead to asymmetric fat distribution with weight gain later in life. Breast asymmetry may occur among females unilaterally irradiated prior to maturity. High doses may stop breast development completely. These effects are decreased or eliminated by reducing radiation doses or fields.

Obesity

Adult survivors of childhood acute lymphoblastic leukemia, particularly females treated at a younger age and previously treated with cranial radiotherapy with cumulative doses of 20 Gy or more have been found to be at a marked increased risk for obesity (Didi et al., 1995; Schell et al., 1992; Van Dongen-Melman et al., 1995; Zee and Chen, 1986). Adult survivors were at two to three times the risk for obesity, relative to sibling controls (i.e., the age- and race-adjusted odds ratio (OR) was 2.59 for females and 1.86 for males). Adult leukemia survivors appear to be more likely to be physically inactive and have reduced exercise capacity, further increasing their risk for obesity (Black et al., 1998; Jenney et al., 1995; Oeffinger et al., 2001; Warner et al., 1998).

A study of both children and adult survivors of ALL found a higher risk of obesity (Mayer et al., 2000). In the cranially irradiated patients, the likely causes of this increased risk included low physical activity, low resting metabolic rate, and hormonal insufficiency.

Interventions to prevent obesity and promote physical activity have been shown to reduce cardiovascular morbidity and mortality and improve quality of life in the general population, and likewise should lower risk in adult survivors. Periodic follow-up to assess weight and physical activity levels and to screen for potential obesity-related diseases is important for adult survivors of childhood cancer, especially those who were treated with cranial irradiation.

Fertility and Reproduction

Treatment with radiation therapy or chemotherapy may have adverse effects on germ cell survival (i.e., ova and sperm), fertility, and the health of offspring (Green et al., 2002a; Green et al., 2002b). Most girls whose entire abdomen or craniospinal area was irradiated fail to enter puberty. Females who maintain or recover ovarian function may enter menopause prematurely. For these women, family planning discussions are important because they may be fertile for only a relatively short period of time. Exposure of the ovary and the dose of radiation affect subsequent ovarian function. Ovarian damage results in both sterilization and loss of hormone production. Ovulating females who receive total body irradiation prior to bone marrow transplantation develop amenorrhea and fewer than 10 percent of women recover normal ovarian function. Reduction in doses of chemotherapeutic agents responsible for ovarian damage has led to improvements in female fertility. Procedures to move the ovaries out of the field of radiation (oophoropexy) have also been used to avoid reproductive late effects.

Males can become infertile following treatment with chemotherapy and radiation, but usually maintain normal hormonal production. Changes in chemotherapy (reduction or elimination of use of alkylating agents) have reduced male infertility following treatment. Sexually mature males about to begin any treatment that could adversely impact fertility should be informed and offered the option of preserving sperm prior to treatment so that the option of artificial insemination is available later.

Hyperprolactinemia, characterized by problems with fertility, growth, and libido, can result after radiation to the hypothalamic-pituitary axis. Some of those treated with high-dose radiotherapy for CNS tumors (not involving the hypothalamic-pituitary axis) were also found to have this hormonal imbalance (Constine et al., 1993; Duffner et al., 1983). Hyperprolactinemia is treatable if identified.

A review of the pregnancy outcomes of female participants in the CCSS showed no adverse outcomes associated with chemotherapeutic agents, but pelvic irradiation increased the risk for low birth weight (Green et al., 2002b). The contribution of somatic or germ cell damage following therapy to the occurrence of low birth weight among offspring of survivors of childhood cancer is not known. Female survivors of Wilms' tumor treated with radiation of the kidney are at increased risk of fetal malposition and premature labor. The offspring of female Wilms' tumor survivors are at risk for low birthweight, premature birth, and the occurrence of congenital malformations (Green et al., 2002a). There were fewer males among the offspring of the partners of the male CCSS participants, as compared with the offspring of the partners of the male siblings, raising the possibility that therapy preferentially interferes with the progression of male fetuses in pregnancies in partners of these survivors (Green et al., 2003 [in press]).

Several recent studies did not identify an increased frequency of major congenital malformations (Byrne et al., 1998; Dodds et al., 1993; Green et al., 1991, 1997; Hawkins, 1991; Janov et al., 1992; Kenney et al., 1996;

Nygaard et al., 1991), genetic disease (Byrne et al., 1998) or childhood cancer (Green et al., 1997; Hawkins et al., 1989; Mulvihill et al., 1987) in the offspring of former pediatric cancer patients, including those conceived after bone marrow transplantation (Sanders et al., 1996), suggesting that the health of offspring appears to be normal.

MUSCULOSKELETAL LATE EFFECTS

Growing children are vulnerable to the effects on their bones of radiation and chemotherapy. Radiation can cause soft tissue hypoplasia (growth impairment), diminution of bone growth, avascular necrosis (circulatory-related tissue damage) (Donaldson and Kaplan, 1982; Libshitz and Edeiken, 1981; Mauch et al., 1983), and epiphyseal slippage (slippage of the bone growth plate) (Dickerman et al., 1979; Silverman et al., 1981). Asymmetric radiation exposure can result in differential growth and lead to functional disabilities, pain, and asymmetric appearance, for example, secondary to scoliosis. These effects of radiation may not be apparent at the end of therapy but emerge with growth, especially during the pubertal growth spurt. Some chemotherapeutic agents (e.g., corticosteroids, methotrexate) also directly affect bone growth. Other agents can indirectly affect growth through damage to hormonal systems (e.g., pituitary-hypothalamic or gonadal dysfunction) (see section above). Treatment regimens for ALL, lymphomas, brain tumors, Wilms' tumor, and sarcomas make survivors particularly vulnerable to these musculoskeletal effects.

Decreased bone mineral density is a multifactorial disorder that is being recognized with increased frequency among survivors of brain tumors (Barr et al., 1998), acute lymphoblastic leukemia (Aisenberg et al., 1998; Arikoski et al., 1998; Nysom et al., 1998), lymphoma (Aisenberg et al., 1998), and solid tumors (Aisenberg et al., 1998). Important risk factors include gonadal dysfunction (Aisenberg et al., 1998), male gender (Arikoski et al., 1998), and prior cranial irradiation (Arikoski et al., 1998; Nysom et al., 1998). Treatment with corticosteroids and methotrexate may impair mineralization (Leiper et al., 1998). These patients may be at increased risk for pathologic fractures as the result of failure to achieve maximal bone mineral accretion during adolescence (Carrascosa et al., 1995). The value of treatment with calcium supplementation, growth hormone, and androgen or estrogen replacement therapy is unknown.

Measures to prevent or reverse bone loss are needed to counter the development of osteoporosis and subsequent bone fractures. Long-term survivors of childhood cancer should be periodically assessed to determine risk for osteoporosis and counseled regarding adequate calcium intake and the benefits of exercise and avoidance of smoking. Exercise, in particular, is known to be effective in increasing bone density among children (Gutin et al., 1999) and young adults (Valdimarsson et al., 1999).

SECOND MALIGNANCIES

The cumulative risk of second malignant cancers 20 years following primary treatment for childhood cancer varies between 3 and 10 percent and is 5 to 20 times greater than that expected in the general population. Radiation therapy is associated with the development of thyroid cancer, breast cancer, melanoma and other skin cancers, brain tumors, and bone and soft tissue sarcomas. Certain types of chemotherapy (i.e., alkylating agents, topoisomerase II inhibitors) are associated with the development of leukemia. Reductions in dose or elimination of radiation for certain embryonal tumors and the reduction in use and alteration in schedule of certain specific drugs may reduce the risk of second malignant cancers. Certain high-risk groups of patients have been identified as those for whom therapy should be modified. An estimated 10 percent of children with ALL, for example, have a defect in a drug-metabolizing enzyme (thiopurine methyltransferase [TPMT]), which places them at increased risk for the development of a second cancer (McLeod et al., 2000).

Women who were treated with chest (mantle) irradiation for childhood Hodgkin's disease face a significant increase in risk for development of breast cancer, with a cumulative incidence of about 35 percent at 20 to 25 years post therapy (Aisenberg et al., 1997; Bhatia et al., 1996). Onset of breast cancer has been noted as early as eight years post radiation, with a median age at diagnosis of 31.5 years (Bhatia et al., 1996) and a median interval from radiation of 15.7 years (Neglia et al., 2001). It appears that pathologic features and prognosis for breast cancer in Hodgkin's survivors are similar to those for the general population (Wolden et al., 2000). Likewise, 5-year survival is strongly associated with stage of disease at time of diagnosis (Cutuli et al., 2001).

There is no consensus about when women who were treated with thoracic radiation therapy should initiate mammographic screening and how frequently they should be screened. The issues surrounding this controversy—usefulness of mammography in dense premenopausal breast, enhancement of breast cancer risk with irradiation exposure by mammography (and the potential for a synergistic effect of irradiation following cancer and its treatment), when to screen girls irradiated in childhood—are areas that require further study.

Children who received radiation or chemotherapeutic agents with known carcinogenic effects should be informed of their risk and should be seen regularly by a health care provider familiar with their treatment and risks who can evaluate early signs and symptoms appropriately. Some survivors of childhood cancers are at increased risk because they have a genetic form of a disease that predisposes them to other cancers. Survivors of the genetic form of retinoblastoma, for example, face risks as high as 50 percent of subsequent secondary cancers over their lifetime. Other rare syndromes predispose survivors to second malignancies (e.g., Li-Fraumeni syndrome, familial polyposis coli).

Skin is sensitive to radiation carcinogenesis, especially at a young age. Doses of radiation used in the treatment of childhood cancers, such as Hodgkin's and non-Hodgkin's lymphomas, soft tissue sarcoma, and Wilms' tumor, are associated with an increased risk for basal cell carcinoma and squamous cell carcinoma (Meadows et al., 1985; Olsen et al., 1993; Swerdlow et al., 1997). Although some follow-up studies of cancer patients have demonstrated an increased risk for malignant melanoma, it is not clear how much, if any, of the excess risk is due to radiation therapy (Shore, 2001). Cancers occur on areas of the skin that were exposed to the radiation. Whether sun protection will lower risk is not known (Lichter et al., 2000; Ron et al., 1991; Ron et al., 1998). However, in recognition of the increased risk for skin cancer after radiation and the benefits of early diagnosis and treatment, it is recommended that health care providers counsel survivors regarding methods of sun protection, the ABCD (Asymmetry, Border, Color, Diameter) rule for early detection of skin cancer, and the importance of periodic examination of the skin in and around the radiation field. Among the general population, public education regarding sun protection and self-examination has been associated with earlier stage of disease at diagnosis (Rhodes, 1995).

OTHER ORGAN DAMAGE

Liver

Because many children with cancer receive blood products during therapy, patients treated before adequate blood donor screening for hepatitis C was initiated in the early 1990s are at risk for chronic liver disease. Estimates of prevalence of exposure to hepatitis C (i.e., as evidenced by presence of hepatitis C viral [HCV] RNA) among ALL and other pediatric cancer patients treated before 1990 ranges from 7 to 49 percent, with an unknown, and likely sizable, percentage of survivors never having been tested or aware of their risk (Dibenedetto et al., 1994; Locasciulli et al., 1997; Paul et al., 1999; Strickland et al., 2000). The health consequences of exposure to hepatitis C among ALL survivors are not well understood. In an Italian study, only two of the 56 HCV-RNA seropositive patients had persistently elevated alanine aminotransferase (ALT) tests for liver inflammation over the course of a mean follow-up of 17 years (Locasciulli and Alberti, 1995). In contrast, Paul et al. reported more serious progression— 12 percent of 75 leukemia survivors were HCV seropositive, 6 of 9 had liver biopsies that showed at least moderate portal inflammation, and half had bridging scarring, consistent with early cirrhosis (Paul et al., 1999).

In the general population, chronic HCV infection develops in 75 to 85 percent of persons infected with hepatitis C (Alter et al., 1992; Shakil et al., 1995). About 30 to 40 percent of chronically infected persons have persistently normal ALT levels and tend to have indolent disease. The course of progressive liver dysfunction is usually insidious, progressing at a slow rate without symptoms or physical signs in the majority of patients during the first two or more decades after infection. Over a 20- to 30-year period, 20 to 30 percent of patients with untreated HCV will develop cirrhosis or extrahepatic sequelae, such as cryoglobulinemia, porphyria cutanea tarda, or membranoproliferative glomerulonephritis (Fattovich et al., 1997; Poynard et al., 1997; Tong et al., 1995). Alcohol consumption, even in moderate amounts, increases the risk of progression to cirrhosis (Pianko et al., 2000; Wiley et al., 1998).

Successful long-term treatment prior to liver decompensation has rapidly improved in the past decade (e.g., treatment with interferon alpha2b and ribavirin) (Lindsay et al., 2001; Poynard et al., 1998). Thus, identification of survivors who were treated with blood products prior to July 1992, determination of their HCV-RNA status, assessment of the liver function of those infected, counseling regarding alcohol consumption, and appropriate treatment and follow-up are essential to reduce the risk for potentially life-threatening sequelae.

Radiation at high doses can also lead to liver damage (e.g., fibrosis).

Kidney and Bladder

Chemotherapy (e.g., cisplatin, ifosfamide), aminoglycoside antibiotics, and some antifungal agents, such as amphotericin B can cause renal failure or damage. Other renal late effects occur secondary to radiation exposure.

Cystitis may occur following treatment with oxazaphosphorine alkylating agents. In one study, the frequency of bladder toxicity was 34 percent among 50 patients treated with pelvic irradiation and cyclophosphamide, compared with 8 percent among 60 patients who received extrapelvic irradiation and cyclophosphamide (Jayalakshmamma and Pinkel, 1976). Medications are now used to protect the bladder from chemotherapy damage, but patients treated before these bladder-protective drugs became available in the late 1990s sometimes sustained damage to the bladder.

Wilms' tumor may be treated by nephrectomy, which sometimes leads to the need for dialysis and transplantation. This occurs rarely and is a greater risk in children with tumors involving both kidneys and those with aniridia or Denys-Drash syndrome (Breslow et al., 2000; Ritchey et al., 1996).

Gastrointestinal

Chemotherapy, radiation therapy, and surgery can contribute to fibrosis (scarring) or inflammation that can interfere with the function of the intestine. Fibrosis and inflammation can also be caused by chronic graft-versus-host disease following allogenic bone marrow transplant. Adhesions, obstructions, ulcers, diarrhea, constipation, and malabsorption can result.

Dental

Radiation therapy that includes the mandible, as for some head and neck cancers and for upper cervical radiation therapy for Hodgkin's disease, can disturb the growth of teeth and affect tooth enamel (e.g., cause pitting) (Jaffe et al., 1984). Dry mouth (xerostomia) due to damage to salivary glands is a common side effect of radiation to the head and neck and medication (Marks et al., 1981; Mira et al., 1981). Lack of saliva predisposes the mouth to oral infection and increases the risk of caries. Administration of amifostine appears to decrease the frequency of chronic xerostomia following irradiation for head and neck cancer (Wasserman et al., 2000). Dry mouth and tooth decay also occur as a consequence of chronic graft-versus-host disease following allogeneic bone marrow transplants.

Sensory Loss

Primary tumors of the CNS, middle ear, and orbital area may be associated with loss of vision and hearing. Radiation therapy may injure the eye lens, retina, or optic nerve and contribute to the formation of cataracts. Prolonged steroid use may also cause cataracts. Hearing loss, which may be reversible, is associated with radiation and long-term administration of several chemotherapies, including cisplatin. The aminoglycoside antibiotics may also produce ototoxicity.

Immune Function

Radiation, chemotherapy, bone marrow transplantation, and removal (or irradiation) of the spleen can impair immune function and decrease the production of blood cells (myelosuppression). The risks of infection among survivors of Hodgkin's disease following removal or irradiation of the spleen are well documented. Children with non-Hodgkin's lymphoma treated with high-dose radiation to the spleen may also face a higher risk of subsequent infections. Total body irradiation prior to bone marrow transplantation may also impair immune system function. In general, the long-term effects of chemotherapy on bone marrow function have not been evaluated exhaustively, but may result in myelosuppression. Administration of the pneumococcal vaccine and the use of prophylactic antibiotics for indefinite periods diminish the risk of infections among those whose spleen has been removed or damaged. Monitoring survivors for immunohematologic dysfunction includes eliciting a detailed history and conducting physical exams for signs and symptoms of recurrent infection, anemia, or bleeding easily.

LATE EFFECTS EMERGING IN ADULTHOOD

Some late effects occur many years after treatment, have an asymptomatic interval, and then become symptomatic only with end-stage or progressive disease, often with devastating consequences. Because the population of adult survivors of childhood cancer is still relatively young, with only a small percentage over the age of 40, very little is known of the eventual effects of cancer and its treatment in older age. Will survivors who experience cognitive dysfunction and neuropathologic changes from cranial irradiation experience premature dementia-type illnesses? Will survivors of soft tissue sarcoma who often experience skeletal problems and asymmetric growth secondary to radiation be at increased risk for premature joint deterioration and chronic muscle spasm and pain? Will clinical or subclinical organ toxicity predispose survivors to premature organ dysfunction/failure? How persistent is the risk of second cancers? Only through long-term follow-up of adult survivors will the impact of these types of late effects on the aging process become evident.

SUMMARY AND CONCLUSIONS

Complications, disabilities, or adverse outcomes that are the result of the disease process, the treatment, or both, are generally referred to as "late effects." Estimates are that as many as two-thirds of survivors will experience a late effect, with perhaps a quarter of survivors experiencing one that is severe or life-threatening. The most common late effects of childhood cancer include those that are neurocognitive and psychological, cardiopulmonary, endocrine (e.g., those affecting growth and fertility), musculoskeletal, and recurrent or second malignancies. The emergence of late effects depends on many factors, including age, exposures to chemotherapy and radiation during treatment (doses and parts of body exposed), and the severity of disease. Complicating the management of late effects is their variable nature. Some may be identified and treated early in follow-up or during the childhood or adolescent years, and resolve without consequence. Others may persist from childhood or arise in adulthood to become chronic problems or influence the progression of other diseases associated with aging. Evidence is lacking for many aspects of care, but does suggest that at least some late effects can be successfully prevented, some can be treated, and others can be managed with expert care.

Assessments of neurocognitive late effects have often been made among ALL survivors. These survivors have a greater likelihood of being placed in special education or learning disabled programs than their siblings, but most are able to compensate and adapt to overcome these problems. Survivors with substantial physical late effects, learning problems, or relapse are more likely than survivors without late effects to show evidence of lower self-esteem, poorer adjustment, and worse quality of life. Some recent research points to psychological problems (Zeltzer et al., 1997) as a result of poor academic achievement secondary to neurocognitive late effects. Psychosocial effects extend to the entire family with recent evidence pointing to significant dysfunction among both siblings and parents of survivors.

The cumulative risk of second malignant cancers 20 years following primary treatment for childhood cancer varies between 3 and 10 percent and is 5 to 20 times greater than that expected in the general population. Despite their increased risks for second cancers, smoking rates among survivors of childhood cancer appear to be equal to those in the general population. Preliminary evidence suggests that there are ways to intervene with tailored smoking cessation interventions in this high-risk population.

Other commonly reported late effects include late-onset cardiac and pulmonary disease among childhood cancer survivors with a history of exposure to certain chemotherapeutic agents (i.e., anthracyclines, notably daunorubicin and doxorubicin) or thoracic radiotherapy; thyroid dysfunction following radiation therapy for Hodgkin's disease, brain tumors, and ALL; alterations in growth and maturation (e.g., growth hormone deficiency, delayed or precocious puberty, hypopituitarism) following cranial irradiation; obesity among survivors of ALL; and fertility problems following radiation therapy or chemotherapy. Not well understood are the consequences of late effects among the aging population of childhood cancer survivors. Research is needed to identify these consequences and effective methods to ameliorate them.

REFERENCES

Abid SH, Malhotra V, Perry MC. 2001. Radiation-induced and chemotherapy-induced pulmonary injury. *Curr Opin Oncol* 13(4):242-8.

Aisenberg AC, Finkelstein DM, Doppke KP, Koerner FC, Boivin JF, Willett CG. 1997. High risk of breast carcinoma after irradiation of young women with Hodgkin's disease. *Cancer* 79(6):1203-10.

Aisenberg J, Hsieh K, Kalaitzoglou G, Whittam E, Heller G, Schneider R, Sklar C. 1998. Bone mineral density in young adult survivors of childhood cancer. *J Pediatr Hematol Oncol* 20(3):241-5.

Alter MJ, Margolis HS, Krawczynski K, Judson FN, Mares A, Alexander WJ, Hu PY, Miller JK, Gerber MA, Sampliner RE, et al. 1992. The natural history of community-acquired hepatitis C in the United States. The Sentinel Counties Chronic non-A, non-B Hepatitis Study Team. *N Engl J Med* 327(27):1899-905.

American Psychiatric Association. 1998. *Diagnostic and Statistical Manual of Mental Disorders*. Amer Psych Assn.

American Cancer Society. 2000. *Cancer Facts and Figures, 2000*. Atlanta, GA: American Cancer Society.

Arikoski P, Komulainen J, Voutilainen R, Riikonen P, Parviainen M, Tapanainen P, Knip M, Kroger H. 1998. Reduced bone mineral density in long-term survivors of childhood acute lymphoblastic leukemia. *J Pediatr Hematol Oncol* 20(3):234-40.

Armstrong FD, Blumberg MJ, Toledano SR. 1999. Neurobehavioral issues in childhood cancer. *School Psychology Review* 28(2):1940-2203.

Arnholt UV, Fritz GK, Keener M. 1993. Self-concept in survivors of childhood and adolescent cancer. *Journal of Psychosocial Oncology* 11(1):1-16.

Barakat LP, Kazak AE, Meadows AT, Casey R, Meeske K, Stuber ML. 1997. Families surviving childhood cancer: a comparison of posttraumatic stress symptoms with families of healthy children. *J Pediatr Psychol* 22(6):843-59.

Barbarin OA, Sargent JR, Sahler OJZ, Carpenter PJ, Copeland DR, Dolgin MJ, Mulhern RK, Roghmann KJ, Zeltzer LK. 1995. Sibling adaptation to childhood cancer collaborative study: Parental views of pre- and postdiagnosis adjustment of siblings of children with cancer. *Journal of Psychosocial Oncology* 13(3):1-20.

Barr RD, Simpson T, Webber CE, Gill GJ, Hay J, Eves M, Whitton AC. 1998. Osteopenia in children surviving brain tumours. *Eur J Cancer* 34(6):873-7.

Bhatia S, Robison LL, Oberlin O, Greenberg M, Bunin G, Fossati-Bellani F, Meadows AT. 1996. Breast cancer and other second neoplasms after childhood Hodgkin's disease. *N Engl J Med* 334(12):745-51.

Black P, Gutjahr P, Stopfkuchen H. 1998. Physical performance in long-term survivors of acute leukaemia in childhood. *Eur J Pediatr* 157(6):464-7.

Breslow NE, Takashima JR, Ritchey ML, Strong LC, Green DM. 2000. Renal failure in the Denys-Drash and Wilms' tumor-aniridia syndromes. *Cancer Res* 60(15):4030-2.

Brouwers P, Neelam J, Krull K, Law R, Fruge E, Bottonley S, Dreyer Z. 2002. Academic and Neurobehavioral Functioning in Long-Term Survivors of Childhood Cancer: Relation to Depression and Anxiety. *Cancer Survivorship: Resilience Across the Lifespan, June 2-4, 2002*. Washington, DC: National Cancer Institute and American Cancer Society.

Butler R, Copeland D, Fairclugh D, Katz E, Kazak A, Mulhern R, Noll R, Sahler OJ. 2002. Neuropsychological Processes and Their Remediation in Children Treated for Cancer. *Cancer Survivorship: Resilience Across the Lifespan, June 2-4, 2002*. Washington, DC: National Cancer Institute and American Cancer Society.

Byrne J, Rasmussen SA, Steinhorn SC, Connelly RR, Myers MH, Lynch CF, Flannery J, Austin DF, Holmes FF, Holmes GE, Strong LC, Mulvihill JJ. 1998. Genetic disease in offspring of long-term survivors of childhood and adolescent cancer. *Am J Hum Genet* 62(1):45-52.

Carlson RG, Mayfield WR, Normann S, Alexander JA. 1991. Radiation-associated valvular disease. *Chest* 99(3):538-45.

Carrascosa A, Gussinye M, Yeste D, del Rio L, Audi L. 1995. Bone mass acquisition during infancy, childhood and adolescence. *Acta Paediatr Suppl* 411:18-23.

Cella DF, Tross S. 1986. Psychological adjustment to survival from Hodgkin's disease. *J Consult Clin Psychol* 54(5):616-22.

Challinor J, Karl D. 1995. Educational attainment in survivors of ALL. *JAMA* 274(14):1134-5.

Chen E, Zeltzer LK, Bentler PM, Byrne J, Nicholson HS, Meadows AT, Mills JL, Haupt R, Fears TR, Robison LL. 1998. Pathways linking treatment intensity and psychosocial outcomes among adult survivors of childhood leukemia. *Journal of Health Psychology* 3(1):23-38.

Chesler M, Barbarin O. 1987. *Childhood Cancer and the Family: Meeting the Challenge of Stress and Support.* New York: Brunner/Mazel.

Clement-De Boers A, Oostdijk W, Van Weel-Sipman MH, Van den Broeck J, Wit JM, Vossen JM. 1996. Final height and hormonal function after bone marrow transplantation in children. *J Pediatr* 129(4):544-50.

Cohen SO, Walco GA. 1999. Dance/movement therapy for children and adolescents with cancer. *Cancer Pract* 7(1):34-42.

Constine LS, Woolf PD, Cann D, Mick G, McCormick K, Raubertas RF, Rubin P. 1993. Hypothalamic-pituitary dysfunction after radiation for brain tumors. *N Engl J Med* 328(2):87-94.

Cutuli B, Borel C, Dhermain F, Magrini SM, Wasserman TH, Bogart JA, Provencio M, de Lafontan B, de la Rochefordiere A, Cellai E, Graic Y, Kerbrat P, Alzieu C, Teissier E, Dilhuydy JM, Mignotte H, Velten M. 2001. Breast cancer occurred after treatment for Hodgkin's disease: analysis of 133 cases. *Radiother Oncol* 59(3):247-55.

DeLaat CA, Lampkin BC. 1992. Long-term survivors of childhood cancer: evaluation and identification of sequelae of treatment. *CA Cancer J Clin* 42(5):263-82.

Dibenedetto SP, Ragusa R, Sciacca A, Di Cataldo A, Miraglia V, D'Amico S, Lo Nigro L, Ippolito AM. 1994. Incidence and morbidity of infection by hepatitis C virus in children with acute lymphoblastic leukaemia. *Eur J Pediatr* 153(4):271-5.

Dickerman JD, Newberg AH, Moreland MD. 1979. Slipped capital femoral epiphysis (SCFE) following pelvic irradiation for rhabdomyosarcoma. *Cancer* 44(2):480-2.

Didi M, Didcock E, Davies HA, Ogilvy-Stuart AL, Wales JK, Shalet SM. 1995. High incidence of obesity in young adults after treatment of acute lymphoblastic leukemia in childhood. *J Pediatr* 127(1):63-7.

Dodds L, Marrett LD, Tomkins DJ, Green B, Sherman G. 1993. Case-control study of congenital anomalies in children of cancer patients. *BMJ* 307(6897):164-8.

Dolgin MJ, Blumensohn R, Mulhern RK, Orbach J, Sahler OJ, Roghmann KJ, Carpenter PJ, Barbarin OA, Sargent JR, Zeltzer LK, Copeland DR. 1997. Sibling Adaptation to Childhood Cancer Collaborative Study: cross-cultural aspects. *Journal of Psychosocial Oncology* 15 (1):1-14.

Donaldson SS. 1993. Lessons from our children. *International Journal of Radiation Oncology, Biology, Physics* 26(5):739-749.

Donaldson SS, Kaplan HS. 1982. Complications of treatment of Hodgkin's disease in children. *Cancer Treat Rep* 66(4):977-89.

Dreyer ZE, Blatt J, Bleyer A. 2002. Late Effects of Childhood Cancer and its Treatment. Pizzo PA, Poplack DG, Eds. *Principles and Practice of Pediatric Oncology.* 4th ed. Philadelphia: Lippincott Williams & Wilkins.

Duffner PK, Cohen ME, Anderson SW, Voorhess ML, MacGillivray MH, Panahon A, Brecher ML. 1983. Long-term effects of treatment on endocrine function in children with brain tumors. *Ann Neurol* 14(5):528-32.

Eiser C, Havermans T. 1994. Long term social adjustment after treatment for childhood cancer. *Archives of Disease in Childhood* 70(1):66-70.

Eiser C, Hill JJ, Vance YH. 2000. Examining the psychological consequences of surviving childhood cancer: systematic review as a research method in pediatric psychology. *J Pediatr Psychol* 25(6):449-60.

Elkin TD, Phipps S, Mulhern RK, Fairclough D. 1997. Psychological functioning of adolescent and young adult survivors of pediatric malignancy. *Med Pediatr Oncol* 29(6): 582-8.

Emmons K, Li FP, Whitton J, Mertens AC, Hutchinson R, Diller L, Robison LL. 2002. Predictors of smoking initiation and cessation among childhood cancer survivors: a report from the childhood cancer survivor study. *J Clin Oncol* 20(6):1608-16.

Exner DV, Dries DL, Waclawiw MA, Shelton B, Domanski MJ. 1999. Beta-adrenergic blocking agent use and mortality in patients with asymptomatic and symptomatic left ventricular systolic dysfunction: a post hoc analysis of the Studies of Left Ventricular Dysfunction. *J Am Coll Cardiol* 33(4):916-23.

Fattovich G, Giustina G, Degos F, Tremolada F, Diodati G, Almasio P, Nevens F, Solinas A, Mura D, Brouwer JT, Thomas H, Njapoum C, Casarin C, Bonetti P, Fuschi P, Basho J, Tocco A, Bhalla A, Galassini R, Noventa F, Schalm SW, Realdi G. 1997. Morbidity and mortality in compensated cirrhosis type C: a retrospective follow-up study of 384 patients. *Gastroenterology* 112(2):463-72.

Fradkin JE, Mills JL, Schonberger LB, Wysowski DK, Thomson R, Durako SJ, Robison LL. 1993. Risk of leukemia after treatment with pituitary growth hormone. *JAMA* 270(23): 2829-32.

Friedman DL, Meadows AT. 2002. Late effects of childhood cancer therapy. *Pediatr Clin North Am* 49(5):1083-106.

Friedrich MJ. 2001. Lowering risk of second malignancy in the survivors of childhood cancer. *JAMA* 285(19):2435-7.

Fritz GK, Williams JR, Amylon M. 1988. After treatment ends: psychosocial sequelae in pediatric cancer survivors. *Am J Orthopsychiatry* 58(4):552-61.

Garre ML, Gandus S, Cesana B, Haupt R, De Bernardi B, Comelli A, Ferrando A, Stella G, Vitali ML, Picco P, et al. 1994. Health status of long-term survivors after cancer in childhood. Results of an uniinstitutional study in Italy. *Am J Pediatr Hematol Oncol* 16(2):143-52.

Ginsberg SJ, Comis RL. 1982. The pulmonary toxicity of antineoplastic agents. *Semin Oncol* 9(1):34-51.

Giorgiani G, Bozzola M, Locatelli F, Picco P, Zecca M, Cisternino M, Dallorso S, Bonetti F, Dini G, Borrone C, et al. 1995. Role of busulfan and total body irradiation on growth of prepubertal children receiving bone marrow transplantation and results of treatment with recombinant human growth hormone. *Blood* 86(2):825-31.

Goldiner PL, Schweizer O. 1979. The hazards of anesthesia and surgery in bleomycin-treated patients. *Semin Oncol* 6(1):121-4.

Goldiner PL, Carlon GC, Cvitkovic E, Schweizer O, Howland WS. 1978. Factors influencing postoperative morbidity and mortality in patients treated with bleomycin. *Br Med J* 1(6128):1664-7.

Gray RE, Doan BD, Shermer P, FitzGerald AV, Berry MP, Jenkin D, Doherty MA. 1992. Psychologic adaptation of survivors of childhood cancer. *Cancer* 70(11):2713-21.

Green DM, Gingell RL, Pearce J, Panahon AM, Ghoorah J. 1987. The effect of mediastinal irradiation on cardiac function of patients treated during childhood and adolescence for Hodgkin's disease. *J Clin Oncol* 5(2):239-45.

Green DM, Zevon MA, Lowrie G, Seigelstein N, Hall B. 1991. Congenital anomalies in children of patients who received chemotherapy for cancer in childhood and adolescence. *N Engl J Med* 325(3):141-6.

Green DM, Fiorello A, Zevon MA, Hall B, Seigelstein N. 1997. Birth defects and childhood cancer in offspring of survivors of childhood cancer. *Arch Pediatr Adolesc Med* 151(4): 379-83.

Green DM, Peabody EM, Nan B, Peterson S, Kalapurakal JA, Breslow NE. 2002a. Pregnancy outcome after treatment for Wilms tumor: a report from the National Wilms Tumor Study Group. *J Clin Oncol* 20(10):2506-13.

Green DM, Whitton JA, Stovall M, Mertens AC, Donaldson SS, Ruymann FB, Pendergrass TW, Robison LL. 2002b. Pregnancy outcome of female survivors of childhood cancer: a report from the Childhood Cancer Survivor Study. *Am J Obstet Gynecol* 187(4): 1070-80.

Green DM, Whitton JA, Stovall M, Mertens AC, Donaldson SS, Ruymann FB, Pendergrass TW, Robison LL. 2003. Pregnancy outcome of partners of male survivors of childhood cancer: a report from the Childhood Cancer Survivor Study. *J Clin Oncol,* Feb. 15; 21(4):716-21.

Greenberg DB, Kornblith AB, Herndon JE, Zuckerman E, Schiffer CA, Weiss RB, Mayer RJ, Wolchok SM, Holland JC. 1997. Quality of life for adult leukemia survivors treated on clinical trials of Cancer and Leukemia Group B during the period 1971-1988: predictors for later psychologic distress. *Cancer* 80(10):1936-44.

Greenberg HS, Kazak AE, Meadows AT. 1989. Psychologic functioning in 8- to 16-year-old cancer survivors and their parents. *J Pediatr* 114(3):488-93.

Grenier MA, Lipshultz SE. 1998. Epidemiology of anthracycline cardiotoxicity in children and adults. *Semin Oncol* 25(4 Suppl 10):72-85.

Gurney JG, Kadan-Lottick NS, Packer RJ, Neglia JP, Sklar CA, Punyko JA, Stovall M, Yasui Y, Nicholson HS, Wolden S, McNeil DE, Mertens AC, Robison LL. 2003. Endocrine and cardiovascular late effects among adult survivors of childhood brain tumors. *Cancer* 97(3):663-73.

Gutin B, Owens S, Okuyama T, Riggs S, Ferguson M, Litaker M. 1999. Effect of physical training and its cessation on percent fat and bone density of children with obesity. *Obes Res* 7(2):208-14.

Haase JE, Rostad M. 1994. Experiences of completing cancer therapy: children's perspectives. *Oncol Nurs Forum* 21(9):1483-92; discussion 1493-4.

Hancock SL, Tucker MA, Hoppe RT. 1993. Breast cancer after treatment of Hodgkin's disease. *J Natl Cancer Inst* 85(1):25-31.

Haupt R, Byrne J, Connelly RR, Mostow EN, Austin DF, Holmes GR, Holmes FF, Latourette HB, Teta MJ, Strong LC, et al. 1992. Smoking habits in survivors of childhood and adolescent cancer. *Med Pediatr Oncol* 20(4):301-6.

Haupt R, Fears TR, Robison LL, Mills JL, Nicholson HS, Zeltzer LK, Meadows AT, Byrne J. 1994. Educational attainment in long-term survivors of childhood acute lymphoblastic leukemia. *JAMA* 272(18):1427-32.

Haupt R, Zeltzer L, Byrne J. 1995. In reply to educational attainment in survivors of ALL. *JAMA* 274(14):1135.

Hawkins MM. 1991. Is there evidence of a therapy-related increase in germ cell mutation among childhood cancer survivors? *J Natl Cancer Inst* 83(22):1643-50.

Hawkins MM, Draper GJ, Smith RA. 1989. Cancer among 1,348 offspring of survivors of childhood cancer. *Int J Cancer* 43(6):975-8.

Hobbie WL, Stuber M, Meeske K, Wissler K, Rourke MT, Ruccione K, Hinkle A, Kazak AE. 2000. Symptoms of posttraumatic stress in young adult survivors of childhood cancer. *J Clin Oncol* 18(24):4060-6.

Hollen PJ. 2000. A clinical profile to predict decision making, risk behaviors, clinical status, and health-related quality of life for cancer-surviving adolescents. Part 1. *Cancer Nurs* 23(4):247-57.

Hollen PJ, Hobbie WL. 1993. Risk taking and decision making of adolescent long-term survivors of cancer. *Oncol Nurs Forum* 20(5):769-76.

Hollen PJ, Hobbie WL. 1996. Decision making and risk behaviors of cancer-surviving adolescents and their peers. *J Pediatr Oncol Nurs* 13(3):121-33; discussion 135-7.

Hollen PJ, Hobbie WL, Finley SM. 1997. Cognitive late effect factors related to decision making and risk behaviors of cancer-surviving adolescents. *Cancer Nurs* 20(5):305-14.

Hollen PJ, Hobbie WL, Finley SM, Hiebert SM. 2001. The relationship of resiliency to decision making and risk behaviors of cancer-surviving adolescents. *J Pediatr Oncol Nurs* 18(5):188-204.

Hovi L, Rajantie J, Perkkio M, Sainio K, Sipila I, Siimes MA. 1990. Growth failure and growth hormone deficiency in children after bone marrow transplantation for leukemia. *Bone Marrow Transplant* 5(3):183-6.

Huma Z, Boulad F, Black P, Heller G, Sklar C. 1995. Growth in children after bone marrow transplantation for acute leukemia. *Blood* 86(2):819-24.

Irwin CE. 1993. Adolescence and risk taking: How are they related? Bell NJ, Bell RW, eds. *Adolescent Risk Taking.*: Newbury Park, CA: Sage Publications. Pp. 1-28.

Iuvone L, Mariotti P, Colosimo C, Guzzetta F, Ruggiero A, Riccardi R. 2002. Long-term cognitive outcome, brain computed tomography scan, and magnetic resonance imaging in children cured for acute lymphoblastic leukemia. *Cancer* 95(12):2562-70.

Jaffe N, Toth BB, Hoar RE, Ried HL, Sullivan MP, McNeese MD. 1984. Dental and maxillofacial abnormalities in long-term survivors of childhood cancer: effects of treatment with chemotherapy and radiation to the head and neck. *Pediatrics* 73(6):816-23.

Janov AJ, Anderson J, Cella DF, Zuckerman E, Kornblith AB, Holland JC, Kantor AF, Li FP, Henderson E, Weiss RB, et al. 1992. Pregnancy outcome in survivors of advanced Hodgkin disease. *Cancer* 70(3):688-92.

Jayalakshmamma B, Pinkel D. 1976. Urinary-bladder toxicity following pelvic irradiation and simultaneous cyclophosphamide therapy. *Cancer* 38(2):701-7.

Jenney ME, Faragher EB, Jones PH, Woodcock A. 1995. Lung function and exercise capacity in survivors of childhood leukaemia. *Med Pediatr Oncol* 24(4):222-30.

Justice B. 1999. Why do women treated for breast cancer report good health despite disease or disability? A pilot study. *Psychol Rep* 84(2):392-4.

Kazak A, Christakis D, Alderfer MCM. 1994. Young adolescent cancer survivors and their parents: adjustments, learning problems, and gender. *Journal of Family Psychology* 8 (1):74-84.

Kazak AE, Meadows AT. 1989. Families of young adolescents who have survived cancer: social-emotional adjustment, adaptability, and social support. *J Pediatr Psychol* 14(2): 175-91.

Kazak AE, Barakat LP, Meeske K, Christakis D, Meadows AT, Casey R, Penati B, Stuber ML. 1997. Posttraumatic stress, family functioning, and social support in survivors of childhood leukemia and their mothers and fathers. *J Consult Clin Psychol* 65(1):120-9.

Kazak AE, Simms S, Barakat L, Hobbie W, Foley B, Golomb V, Best M. 1999. Surviving cancer competently intervention program (SCCIP): a cognitive-behavioral and family therapy intervention for adolescent survivors of childhood cancer and their families. *Fam Process* 38(2):175-91.

Kazak AE, Alderfer M, Rourke M, Simms S, Streisand R. 2002. Posttraumatic Stress in Adolescent Survivors of Childhood Cancer and Their Mothers, Father, and Siblings, Poster Presentation. *Cancer Survivorship: Resilience Across the Lifespan, June 2-4, 2002.* Washington, DC: National Cancer Institute and American Cancer Society.

Keene N, Hobbie W, Ruccione K. 2000. *Childhood Cancer Survivors: A Practical Guide to Your Future.* Sebastopol, CA: O'Reilly and Associates, Inc.

Kenney LB, Nicholson HS, Brasseux C, Mills JL, Robison LL, Zeltzer LK, Meadows AT, Reaman GH, Byrne J. 1996. Birth defects in offspring of adult survivors of childhood acute lymphoblastic leukemia. A Childrens Cancer Group/National Institutes of Health Report. *Cancer* 78(1):169-76.

Kingma A, van Dommelen RI, Mooyaart EL, Wilmink JT, Deelman BG, Kamps WA. 2001. Slight cognitive impairment and magnetic resonance imaging abnormalities but normal school levels in children treated for acute lymphoblastic leukemia with chemotherapy only. *J Pediatr* 139(3):413-20.

Koocher GP, O'Malley JE. 1981. *The Damocles Syndrome: Psychosocial Consequences of Surviving Childhood Cancer.* New York: McGraw-Hill.

Koocher GP, O'Malley JE, Gogan JL, Foster DJ. 1980. Psychological adjustment among pediatric cancer survivors. *Journal of Child Psychology & Psychiatry & Allied Disciplines* 21(2):163-73.

Kornblith AB, Herndon JE 2nd, Zuckerman E, Cella DF, Cherin E, Wolchok S, Weiss RB, Diehl LF, Henderson E, Cooper MR, Schiffer C, Canellos GP, Mayer RJ, Silver RT, Schilling A, Peterson BA, Greenberg D, Holland JC. 1998. Comparison of psychosocial adaptation of advanced stage Hodgkin's disease and acute leukemia survivors. Cancer and Leukemia Group B. *Ann Oncol* 9(3):297-306.

Kupst MJ, Schulman JL. 1988. Long-term coping with pediatric leukemia: a six-year follow-up study. *J Pediatr Psychol* 13(1):7-22.

Kupst MJ, Natta MB, Richardson CC, Schulman JL, Lavigne JV, Das L. 1995. Family coping with pediatric leukemia: ten years after treatment. *J Pediatr Psychol* 20(5):601-17.

Lansky SB, List MA, Ritter-Sterr C. 1986. Psychosocial consequences of cure. *Cancer* 58(2 Suppl):529-33.

Leiper AD, Stanhope R, Lau T, Grant DB, Blacklock H, Chessells JM, Plowman PN. 1987. The effect of total body irradiation and bone marrow transplantation during childhood and adolescence on growth and endocrine function. *Br J Haematol* 67(4):419-26.

Leonard GT, Green DM, Spengenthal EL, et al. 2000. Cardiac mortality and morbidity after treatment for Hodgkin disease during childhood or adolescence. *Pediatrc Res* 47(46A).

Libshitz HI, Edeiken BS. 1981. Radiotherapy changes of the pediatric hip. *AJR Am J Roentgenol* 137(3):585-8.

Lichter MD, Karagas MR, Mott LA, Spencer SK, Stukel TA, Greenberg ER. 2000. Therapeutic ionizing radiation and the incidence of basal cell carcinoma and squamous cell carcinoma. The New Hampshire Skin Cancer Study Group. *Arch Dermatol* 136(8):1007-11.

Lindsay KL, Trepo C, Heintges T, Shiffman ML, Gordon SC, Hoefs JC, Schiff ER, Goodman ZD, Laughlin M, Yao R, Albrecht JK. 2001. A randomized, double-blind trial comparing pegylated interferon alfa-2b to interferon alfa-2b as initial treatment for chronic hepatitis C. *Hepatology* 34(2):395-403.

Lipshultz SE, Colan SD, Gelber RD, Perez-Atayde AR, Sallan SE, Sanders SP. 1991. Late cardiac effects of doxorubicin therapy for acute lymphoblastic leukemia in childhood. *N Engl J Med* 324(12):808-15.

Lipshultz SE, Lipsitz SR, Mone SM, Goorin AM, Sallan SE, Sanders SP, Orav EJ, Gelber RD, Colan SD. 1995. Female sex and drug dose as risk factors for late cardiotoxic effects of doxorubicin therapy for childhood cancer. *N Engl J Med* 332(26):1738-43.

Locasciulli A, Alberti A. 1995. Hepatitis C virus serum markers and liver disease in children with leukemia. *Leuk Lymphoma* 17(3-4):245-9.

Locasciulli A, Testa M, Pontisso P, Benvegnu L, Fraschini D, Corbetta A, Noventa F, Masera G, Alberti A. 1997. Prevalence and natural history of hepatitis C infection in patients cured of childhood leukemia. *Blood* 90(11):4628-33.

Mackie E, Hill J, Kondryn H, McNally R. 2000. Adult psychosocial outcomes in long-term survivors of acute lymphoblastic leukaemia and Wilms' tumour: a controlled study. *Lancet* 355(9212):1310-4.

Maggiolini A, Grassi R, Adamoli L, Corbetta A, Charmet GP, Provantini K, Fraschini D, Jankovic M, Lia R, Spinetta J, Masera G. 2000. Self-image of adolescent survivors of long-term childhood leukemia. *J Pediatr Hematol Oncol* 22(5):417-21.

Marina N. 1997. Long-term survivors of childhood cancer. The medical consequences of cure. *Pediatr Clin North Am* 44(4):1021-42.

Marks JE, Davis CC, Gottsman VL, Purdy JE, Lee F. 1981. The effects of radiation on parotid salivary function. *Int J Radiat Oncol Biol Phys* 7(8):1013-9.

Mauch PM, Weinstein H, Botnick L, Belli J, Cassady JR. 1983. An evaluation of long-term survival and treatment complications in children with Hodgkin's disease. *Cancer* 51(5): 925-32.

Mayer EI, Reuter M, Dopfer RE, Ranke MB. 2000. Energy expenditure, energy intake and prevalence of obesity after therapy for acute lymphoblastic leukemia during childhood. *Horm Res* 53(4):193-9.

McKelvie RS, Benedict CR, Yusuf S. 1999. Evidence based cardiology: prevention of congestive heart failure and management of asymptomatic left ventricular dysfunction. *BMJ* 318(7195):1400-2.

McLeod HL, Krynetski EY, Relling MV, Evans WE. 2000. Genetic polymorphism of thiopurine methyltransferase and its clinical relevance for childhood acute lymphoblastic leukemia. *Leukemia* 14(4):567-72.

Meadows AT, Baum E, Fossati-Bellani F, Green D, Jenkin RD, Marsden B, Nesbit M, Newton W, Oberlin O, Sallan SG, et al. 1985. Second malignant neoplasms in children: an update from the Late Effects Study Group. *J Clin Oncol* 3(4):532-8.

Meeske KA, Ruccione K, Globe DR, Stuber ML. 2001. Posttraumatic stress, quality of life, and psychological distress in young adult survivors of childhood cancer. *Oncol Nurs Forum* 28(3):481-9.

Meister LA, Meadows AT. 1993. Late effects of childhood cancer therapy. *Curr Probl Pediatr* 23(3):102-31.

Mertens AC, Yasui Y, Neglia JP, Potter JD, Nesbit ME Jr, Ruccione K, Smithson WA, Robison LL. 2001. Late mortality experience in five-year survivors of childhood and adolescent cancer: the Childhood Cancer Survivor Study. *J Clin Oncol* 19(13):3163-72.

Mertens AC, Yasui Y, Liu Y, Stovall M, Hutchinson R, Ginsberg J, Sklar C, Robison LL. 2002. Pulmonary complications in survivors of childhood and adolescent cancer. A report from the Childhood Cancer Survivor Study. *Cancer* 95(11):2431-41.

Mira JG, Wescott WB, Starcke EN, Shannon IL. 1981. Some factors influencing salivary function when treating with radiotherapy. *Int J Radiat Oncol Biol Phys* 7(4):535-41.

Moller TR, Garwicz S, Barlow L, Falck Winther J, Glattre E, Olafsdottir G, Olsen JH, Perfekt R, Ritvanen A, Sankila R, Tulinius H. 2001. Decreasing late mortality among five-year survivors of cancer in childhood and adolescence: a population-based study in the Nordic countries. *J Clin Oncol* 19(13):3173-81.

Moore I, Glasser M, Ablin A. 1987. Late psychosocial consequences of childhood cancer. *Journal of Pediatric Nursing* 3(3):150.

Mulhern RK, Wasserman AL, Fairclough D, Ochs J. 1988. Memory function in disease-free survivors of childhood acute lymphocytic leukemia given CNS prophylaxis with or without 1,800 cGy cranial irradiation. *J Clin Oncol* 6(2):315-20.

Mulhern RK, Wasserman AL, Friedman AG, Fairclough D. 1989. Social competence and behavioral adjustment of children who are long-term survivors of cancer. *Pediatrics* 83(1):18-25.

Mulhern RK, Tyc VL, Phipps S, Crom D, Barclay D, Greenwald C, Hudson M, Thompson EI. 1995. Health-related behaviors of survivors of childhood cancer. *Med Pediatr Oncol* 25(3):159-65.

Mulvihill JJ, Myers MH, Connelly RR, Byrne J, Austin DF, Bragg K, Cook JW, Hassinger DD, Holmes FF, Holmes GF, et al. 1987. Cancer in offspring of long-term survivors of childhood and adolescent cancer. *Lancet* 2(8563):813-7.

Neglia JP, Nesbit ME Jr. 1993. Care and treatment of long-term survivors of childhood cancer. *Cancer* 71(10 Suppl):3386-91.

Neglia JP, Friedman DL, Yasui Y, Mertens AC, Hammond S, Stovall M, Donaldson SS, Meadows AT, Robison LL. 2001. Second malignant neoplasms in five-year survivors of childhood cancer: Childhood Cancer Survivor Study. *J Natl Cancer Inst* 93(8):618-29.

Nolen-Hoeksema S. 1987. Sex differences in unipolar depression: evidence and theory. *Psychological Bulletin* 101(2):259-82.

Noll RB, MacLean WE Jr, Whitt JK, Kaleita TA, Stehbens JA, Waskerwitz MJ, Ruymann FB, Hammond GD. 1997. Behavioral adjustment and social functioning of long-term survivors of childhood leukemia: parent and teacher reports. *J Pediatr Psychol* 22(6):827-41.

Nygaard R, Clausen N, Siimes MA, Marky I, Skjeldestad FE, Kristinsson JR, Vuoristo A, Wegelius R, Moe PJ. 1991. Reproduction following treatment for childhood leukemia: a population-based prospective cohort study of fertility and offspring. *Med Pediatr Oncol* 19(6):459-66.

Nysom K, Holm K, Michaelsen KF, Hertz H, Muller J, Molgaard C. 1998. Bone mass after treatment for acute lymphoblastic leukemia in childhood. *J Clin Oncol* 16(12):3752-60.

O'Driscoll BR, Hasleton PS, Taylor PM, Poulter LW, Gattameneni HR, Woodcock AA. 1990. Active lung fibrosis up to 17 years after chemotherapy with carmustine (BCNU) in childhood. *N Engl J Med* 323(6):378-82.

O'Driscoll BR, Kalra S, Gattamaneni HR, Woodcock AA. 1995. Late carmustine lung fibrosis. Age at treatment may influence severity and survival. *Chest* 107(5):1355-7.

Oberfield SE, Sklar CA. 2002. Endocrine sequelae in survivors of childhood cancer. *Adolesc Med* 13(1):161-9, viii.

Ochs J, Mulhern R, Fairclough D, Parvey L, Whitaker J, Ch'ien L, Mauer A, Simone J. 1991. Comparison of neuropsychologic functioning and clinical indicators of neurotoxicity in long-term survivors of childhood leukemia given cranial radiation or parenteral methotrexate: a prospective study. *J Clin Oncol* 9(1):145-51.

Oeffinger KC, Eshelman DA, Tomlinson GE, Buchanan GR, Foster BM. 2000. Grading of late effects in young adult survivors of childhood cancer followed in an ambulatory adult setting. *Cancer* 88(7):1687-95.

Oeffinger KC, Buchanan GR, Eshelman DA, Denke MA, Andrews TC, Germak JA, Tomlinson GE, Snell LE, Foster BM. 2001. Cardiovascular risk factors in young adult survivors of childhood acute lymphoblastic leukemia. *J Pediatr Hematol Oncol* 23(7):424-30.

Olsen JH, Garwicz S, Hertz H, Jonmundsson G, Langmark F, Lanning M, Lie SO, Moe PJ, Moller T, Sankila R, et al. 1993. Second malignant neoplasms after cancer in childhood or adolescence. Nordic Society of Paediatric Haematology and Oncology Association of the Nordic Cancer Registries. *BMJ* 307(6911):1030-6.

Packer RJ, Meadows AT, Rorke LB, Goldwein JL, D'Angio G. 1987. Long-term sequelae of cancer treatment on the central nervous system in childhood. *Med Pediatr Oncol* 15(5): 241-53.

Papadimitriou A, Urena M, Hamill G, Stanhope R, Leiper AD. 1991. Growth hormone treatment of growth failure secondary to total body irradiation and bone marrow transplantation. *Arch Dis Child* 66(6):689-92.

Paul IM, Sanders J, Ruggiero F, Andrews T, Ungar D, Eyster ME. 1999. Chronic hepatitis C virus infections in leukemia survivors: prevalence, viral load, and severity of liver disease. *Blood* 93(11):3672-7.

Pianko S, Patella S, Sievert W. 2000. Alcohol consumption induces hepatocyte apoptosis in patients with chronic hepatitis C infection. *J Gastroenterol Hepatol* 15(7):798-805.

Poynard T, Bedossa P, Opolon P. 1997. Natural history of liver fibrosis progression in patients with chronic hepatitis C. The OBSVIRC, METAVIR, CLINIVIR, and DOSVIRC groups. *Lancet* 349(9055):825-32.

Poynard T, Marcellin P, Lee SS, Niederau C, Minuk GS, Ideo G, Bain V, Heathcote J, Zeuzem S, Trepo C, Albrecht J. 1998. Randomised trial of interferon alpha2b plus ribavirin for 48 weeks or for 24 weeks versus interferon alpha2b plus placebo for 48 weeks for treatment of chronic infection with hepatitis C virus. International Hepatitis Interventional Therapy Group (IHIT). *Lancet* 352(9138):1426-32.

Prasad VK, Lewis IJ, Aparicio SR, Heney D, Hale JP, Bailey CC, Kinsey SE. 1996. Progressive glomerular toxicity of ifosfamide in children. *Med Pediatr Oncol* 27(3):149-55.

Probert JC, Parker BR. 1975. The effects of radiation therapy on bone growth. *Radiology* 114(1):155-62.

Rait DS, Ostroff JS, Smith K, Cella DF, Tan C, Lesko LM. 1992. Lives in a balance: perceived family functioning and the psychosocial adjustment of adolescent cancer survivors. *Fam Process* 31(4):383-97.

Rauck AM, Green DM, Yasui Y, Mertens A, Robison LL. 1999. Marriage in the survivors of childhood cancer: a preliminary description from the Childhood Cancer Survivor Study. *Med Pediatr Oncol* 33(1):60-3.

Rhodes AR. 1995. Public education and cancer of the skin. What do people need to know about melanoma and nonmelanoma skin cancer? *Cancer* 75(2 Suppl):613-36.

Riseborough EJ, Grabias SL, Burton RI, Jaffe N. 1976. Skeletal alterations following irradiation for Wilms' tumor: with particular reference to scoliosis and kyphosis. *J Bone Joint Surg Am* 58(4):526-36.

Ritchey ML, Green DM, Thomas PR, Smith GR, Haase G, Shochat S, Moksness J, Breslow NE. 1996. Renal failure in Wilms' tumor patients: a report from the National Wilms' Tumor Study Group. *Med Pediatr Oncol* 26(2):75-80.

Roberts CS, Turney ME, Knowles AM. 1998. Psychosocial issues of adolescents with cancer. *Soc Work Health Care* 27(4):3-18.

Ron E, Modan B, Preston D, Alfandary E, Stovall M, Boice JD Jr. 1991. Radiation-induced skin carcinomas of the head and neck. *Radiat Res* 125(3):318-25.

Ron E, Preston DL, Kishikawa M, Kobuke T, Iseki M, Tokuoka S, Tokunaga M, Mabuchi K. 1998. Skin tumor risk among atomic-bomb survivors in Japan. *Cancer Causes Control* 9(4):393-401.

Rourke MT, Stuber ML, Hobbie WL, Kazak AE. 1999. Posttraumatic stress disorder: understanding the psychosocial impact of surviving childhood cancer into young adulthood. *J Pediatr Oncol Nurs* 16(3):126-35.

Rubenstein CL, Varni JW, Katz ER. 1990. Cognitive functioning in long-term survivors of childhood leukemia: a prospective analysis. *J Dev Behav Pediatr* 11(6):301-5.

Sahler OJ, Roghmann KJ, Carpenter PJ, Mulhern RK, Dolgin MJ, Sargent JR, Barbarin OA, Copeland DR, Zeltzer LK. 1994. Sibling adaptation to childhood cancer collaborative study: prevalence of sibling distress and definition of adaptation levels. *J Dev Behav Pediatr* 15(5):353-66.

Sanders JE, Pritchard S, Mahoney P, Amos D, Buckner CD, Witherspoon RP, Deeg HJ, Doney KC, Sullivan KM, Appelbaum FR, et al. 1986. Growth and development following marrow transplantation for leukemia. *Blood* 68(5):1129-35.

Sanders JE, Hawley J, Levy W, Gooley T, Buckner CD, Deeg HJ, Doney K, Storb R, Sullivan K, Witherspoon R, Appelbaum FR. 1996. Pregnancies following high-dose cyclophosphamide with or without high-dose busulfan or total-body irradiation and bone marrow transplantation. *Blood* 87(7):3045-52.

Sargent JR, Sahler OJ, Roghmann KJ, Mulhern RK, Barbarian OA, Carpenter PJ, Copeland DR, Dolgin MJ, Zeltzer LK. 1995. Sibling adaptation to childhood cancer collaborative study: siblings' perceptions of the cancer experience. *J Pediatr Psychol* 20(2):151-64.

Schell MJ, Ochs JJ, Schriock EA, Carter M. 1992. A method of predicting adult height and obesity in long-term survivors of childhood acute lymphoblastic leukemia. *J Clin Oncol* 10(1):128-33.

Schwartz C, Hobbie W, Constine L, Ruccione K. 1994. *Survivors of Childhood Cancer: Assessment and Management.* St. Louis, MO: Mosby.

Schwartz CL. 1995. Late effects of treatment in long-term survivors of cancer. *Cancer Treat Rev* 21(4):355-66.

Schwartz CL. 1999. Long-term survivors of childhood cancer: the late effects of therapy. *Oncologist* 4(1):45-54.

Shakil AO, Conry-Cantilena C, Alter HJ, Hayashi P, Kleiner DE, Tedeschi V, Krawczynski K, Conjeevaram HS, Sallie R, Di Bisceglie AM. 1995. Volunteer blood donors with antibody to hepatitis C virus: clinical, biochemical, virologic, and histologic features. The Hepatitis C Study Group. *Ann Intern Med* 123(5):330-7.

Shan K, Lincoff AM, Young JB. 1996. Anthracycline-induced cardiotoxicity. *Ann Intern Med* 125(1):47-58.

Shore RE. 2001. Radiation-induced skin cancer in humans. *Med Pediatr Oncol* 36(5):549-54.

Silverman CL, Thomas PR, McAlister WH, Walker S, Whiteside LA. 1981. Slipped femoral capital epiphyses in irradiated children: dose, volume and age relationships. *Int J Radiat Oncol Biol Phys* 7(10):1357-63.

Skinner R, Cotterill SJ, Stevens MC. 2000. Risk factors for nephrotoxicity after ifosfamide treatment in children: a UKCCSG Late Effects Group study. United Kingdom Children's Cancer Study Group. *Br J Cancer* 82(10):1636-45.

Sklar C, Whitton J, Mertens A, Stovall M, Green D, Marina N, Greffe B, Wolden S, Robison L. 2000. Abnormalities of the thyroid in survivors of Hodgkin's disease: data from the Childhood Cancer Survivor Study. *J Clin Endocrinol Metab* 85(9):3227-32.

Sklar CA, Mertens AC, Mitby P, Occhiogrosso G, Qin J, Heller G, Yasui Y, Robison LL. 2002. Risk of disease recurrence and second neoplasms in survivors of childhood cancer treated with growth hormone: a report from the Childhood Cancer Survivor Study. *J Clin Endocrinol Metab* 87(7):3136-41.

Smith MA, Ries LAG. 2002. Childhood Cancer: Incidence, Survival, and Mortality. Pizzo PA, Poplack DG, Eds. *Principles and Practice of Pediatric Oncology.* 4th ed. Philadelphia: Lippincott Williams & Wilkins.

Steinherz LJ, Steinherz PG, Tan CT, Heller G, Murphy ML. 1991. Cardiac toxicity 4 to 20 years after completing anthracycline therapy. *JAMA* 266(12):1672-7.

Stevens MC, Mahler H, Parkes S. 1998. The health status of adult survivors of cancer in childhood. *Eur J Cancer* 34(5):694-8.

Strickland DK, Riely CA, Patrick CC, Jones-Wallace D, Boyett JM, Waters B, Fleckenstein JF, Dean PJ, Davila R, Caver TE, Hudson MM. 2000. Hepatitis C infection among survivors of childhood cancer. *Blood* 95(10):3065-70.

Stuber ML, Christakis DA, Houskamp B, Kazak AE. 1996. Posttrauma symptoms in childhood leukemia survivors and their parents. *Psychosomatics* 37(3):254-61.

Swerdlow AJ, Barber JA, Horwich A, Cunningham D, Milan S, Omar RZ. 1997. Second malignancy in patients with Hodgkin's disease treated at the Royal Marsden Hospital. Br J Cancer 75(1):116-23.

Tao ML, Guo MD, Weiss R, Byrne J, Mills JL, Robison LL, Zeltzer LK. 1998. Smoking in adult survivors of childhood acute lymphoblastic leukemia. J Natl Cancer Inst 90(3):219-25.

Tong MJ, el-Farra NS, Reikes AR, Co RL. 1995. Clinical outcomes after transfusion-associated hepatitis C. N Engl J Med 332(22):1463-6.

Troyer H, Holmes G. 1988. Cigarette smoking among childhood cancer survivors. American Journal of Disease of Childhood 142:123.

Valdimarsson O, Kristinsson JO, Stefansson SO, Valdimarsson S, Sigurdsson G. 1999. Lean mass and physical activity as predictors of bone mineral density in 16-20-year old women. J Intern Med 245(5):489-96.

Van Dongen-Melman JE. 2000. Developing psychosocial aftercare for children surviving cancer and their families. Acta Oncol 39(1):23-31.

Van Dongen-Melman JE, Sanders-Woudstra JA. 1986. Psychosocial aspects of childhood cancer: a review of the literature. J Child Psychol Psychiatry 27(2):145-80.

Van Dongen-Melman JE, Hokken-Koelega AC, Hahlen K, De Groot A, Tromp CG, Egeler RM. 1995. Obesity after successful treatment of acute lymphoblastic leukemia in childhood. Pediatr Res 38(1):86-90.

Vonderweid N, Beck D, Caflisch U, Feldges A, Wyss M, Wagner HP. 1996. Standardized assessment of late effects in long-term survivors of childhood cancer in Switzerland: results of a Swiss Pediatric Oncology Group (SPOG) pilot study. International Journal of Pediatric Hematology/Oncology 3:483.

Waber DP, Carpentieri SC, Klar N, Silverman LB, Schwenn M, Hurwitz CA, Mullenix PJ, Tarbell NJ, Sallan SE. 2000. Cognitive sequelae in children treated for acute lymphoblastic leukemia with dexamethasone or prednisone. J Pediatr Hematol Oncol 22(3):206-13.

Walker C. 1989. Use of art and play therapy in pediatric oncology. J Pediatr Oncol Nurs 6(4):121-6.

Ward, JD. 2000. Pediatric cancer survivors: assessment of late effects. Nurse Pract. 25(12):18, 21-8, 35-7; quiz 38-9.

Warner JT, Bell W, Webb DK, Gregory JW. 1998. Daily energy expenditure and physical activity in survivors of childhood malignancy. Pediatr Res 43(5):607-13.

Wasserman AL, Thompson EI, Wilimas JA, Fairclough DL. 1987. The psychological status of survivors of childhood/adolescent Hodgkin's disease. American Journal of Diseases of Children 141(6):626-31.

Wasserman T, Mackowiak JI, Brizel DM, Oster W, Zhang J, Peeples PJ, Sauer R. 2000. Effect of amifostine on patient assessed clinical benefit in irradiated head and neck cancer. Int J Radiat Oncol Biol Phys 48(4):1035-9.

Weigers ME, Chesler MA, Zebrack BJGS. 1998. Self-reported worries among long-term survivors of chilodhood cancer and their peers. Journal of Psyhosocial Oncology 16(2):1-24.

Wexler LH. 1998. Ameliorating anthracycline cardiotoxicity in children with cancer: clinical trials with dexrazoxane. Semin Oncol 25(4 Suppl 10):86-92.

Wiley TE, McCarthy M, Breidi L, McCarthy M, Layden TJ. 1998. Impact of alcohol on the histological and clinical progression of hepatitis C infection. Hepatology 28(3):805-9.

Wingard JR, Plotnick LP, Freemer CS, Zahurak M, Piantadosi S, Miller DF, Vriesendorp HM, Yeager AM, Santos GW. 1992. Growth in children after bone marrow transplantation: busulfan plus cyclophosphamide versus cyclophosphamide plus total body irradiation. Blood 79(4):1068-73.

Wolden SL, Hancock SL, Carlson RW, Goffinet DR, Jeffrey SS, Hoppe RT. 2000. Management of breast cancer after Hodgkin's disease. *J Clin Oncol* 18(4):765-72.

Zebrack BJ, Chesler MA. 2002. Quality of life in childhood cancer survivors. *Psychooncology* 11(2):132-41.

Zebrack BJ, Zeltzer LK, Whitton J, Mertens AC, Odom L, Berkow R, Robison LL. 2002. Psychological outcomes in long-term survivors of childhood leukemia, Hodgkin's disease, and non-Hodgkin's lymphoma: a report from the Childhood Cancer Survivor Study. *Pediatrics* 110(1 Pt 1):42-52.

Zee P, Chen CH. 1986. Prevalence of obesity in children after therapy for acute lymphoblastic leukemia. *Am J Pediatr Hematol Oncol* 8(4):294-9.

Zeltzer LK. 1993. Cancer in adolescents and young adults psychosocial aspects. Long-term survivors. *Cancer* 71(10 Suppl):3463-8.

Zeltzer LK, Dolgin MJ, Sahler OJ, Roghmann K, Barbarin OA, Carpenter PJ, Copeland DR, Mulhern RK, Sargent JR. 1996. Sibling adaptation to childhood cancer collaborative study: health outcomes of siblings of children with cancer. *Med Pediatr Oncol* 27(2):98-107.

Zeltzer LK, Chen E, Weiss R, Guo MD, Robison LL, Meadows AT, Mills JL, Nicholson HS, Byrne J. 1997. Comparison of psychologic outcome in adult survivors of childhood acute lymphoblastic leukemia versus sibling controls: a cooperative Children's Cancer Group and National Institutes of Health study. *J Clin Oncol* 15(2):547-56.

5

Delivering Survivorship Care

Increased recognition of cancer's late effects has meant that some childhood cancer survivors have joined the ranks of the relatively large group of children with chronic conditions and ongoing health problems. This chapter first reviews the current status of pediatric cancer care—both initial treatment and follow-up care—in terms of where care is provided, who provides care, and how care is paid for. Next, similarities and differences are drawn between the long-term health care needs of cancer survivors and other children with chronic illness or disabilities. Finally, the components of an ideal care system designed to meet the unique continuing health care needs of childhood cancer survivors are described and the relative strengths and limitations of alternate delivery models for follow-up care are outlined.

CURRENT STATUS OF PEDIATRIC CANCER CARE

Childhood cancer is rare and therefore accounts for a relatively small share of health care. An estimated 3 per 1,000 pediatric ambulatory visits and an equal share of pediatric hospitalizations are for the care of patients under age 20 with cancer (Table 5.1). Each year there are an estimated 605,600 cancer-related ambulatory care visits and 20,590 hospital discharges among children (Table 5.1). These estimates from large national surveys and administrative data sets pertain to the entire spectrum of cancer care, from diagnosis and treatment to end-of-life care. Pediatric cancer care, once offered predominantly in hospitals, has increasingly been provided on an outpatient basis (Mullen et al., 1999; Wolfe, 1993; Wollnik, 1976).

Pediatric cancer care also appears to be concentrated in specialty settings—nearly half (46 percent) of cancer-related ambulatory care is provided in hospital-based outpatient clinics and 58 percent of cancer-related hospital care takes place in urban, teaching hospitals (Table 5.1).

The implications of uninsuredness for children with cancer are dire given the complexity of care and its associated costs. An estimated 7 percent of cancer-related ambulatory care visits made from 1995 to 1999 by children were not covered by insurance, and 3 percent of cancer-related hospital discharges in 1997 lacked coverage (Table 5.1). Coverage of cancer-related ambulatory care visits is primarily through private insurance (62 percent) and to a lesser extent the Medicaid program (6 percent) (Table 5.1). Cancer-related hospital care is more heavily dependent on public programs—31 percent of hospitalizations were paid for by the Medicaid program and 60 percent were paid for by private insurance in 1997 (Table 5.1). Some low-income individuals and families who lack health insurance, but who are not eligible for Medicaid, "spend down" to become eligible for Medicaid to help pay for expensive hospitalizations. Pediatric cancer care tends to be intensive, lengthy, and costly. An estimated 18 percent of cancer-related hospitalizations had length of stays of 14 or more days (National Cancer Policy Board [NCPB] special tabulations). Total charges associated with cancer-related hospital care are very high; 22 percent of discharges had total charges of $40,000 and above in 1997 (NCPB special tabulations).

There have been relatively few studies of the costs associated with caring for children with cancer, but one study conducted in the early 1980s suggests that family out-of-pocket expenses add about 50 percent to the total cost of disease-related care and consumed 38 percent of gross annual family income (Bloom et al., 1985). Not measured are the broader costs incurred by the family, including lost wages and opportunity costs (e.g., lack of job advancement).

Initial Treatment of Childhood Cancer:
The Intersection of Cancer Care and Research

It is generally recognized that children undergoing their initial treatment for cancer and their families have special needs that can best be met by specialized children's cancer centers. Such centers use a team approach involving a variety of specialists— pediatric oncologists, surgeons, radiation oncologists, pediatric oncology nurses, nurse practitioners, psychologists, social workers, child life specialists, nutritionists, rehabilitation and physical therapists, and educators—who can support and educate the entire family. In recognition of improved outcomes associated with such specialized care, the American Academy of Pediatrics (AAP) recommends that

TABLE 5.1 Estimates of the Number and Distribution of Cancer-Related
Pediatric Ambulatory Care Visits and Hospital Discharges, by Age, Sex,
Race/Ethnicity, Payment, and Site of Care, NAMCS and NHAMCS,
1995-1999, HCUP NIS, 1997

Characteristic	Ambulatory Visits		Hospital Discharges	
	Annual population estimate[a]	% (se)	Annual population estimate[a]	% (se)
Total	605,600	100.0	20,590	100.0
Age				
0	44,600	7.4 (2.0)	930	4.5 (0.5)
1-4	161,500	26.7 (3.4)	5,170	25.1 (1.1)
5-9	126,600	20.9 (3.1)	5,190	25.2 (1.0)
10-14	154,900	25.6 (3.4)	4,210	20.4 (0.9)
15-19	117,900	19.5 (3.1)	5,090	24.7 (1.8)
Sex				
Male	377,000	62.3 (3.7)	11,690	56.8 (1.1)
Female	228,500	37.7 (3.7)	8,890	43.2 (1.1)
Race/ethnicity[b]				
White, non-Hispanic	437,400	72.2 (3.5)	10,100	65.7 (3.6)
White, Hispanic	98,700	16.3 (2.8)	2,300	15.0 (2.9)
African American	34,300	5.7 (1.8)	1,920	12.5 (1.6)
Other	35,200	5.8 (1.8)	1,040	6.8 (1.7)

children and adolescents with newly diagnosed or recurrent malignancies
receive their treatment in a pediatric cancer center (American Academy of
Pediatrics, 1997). The AAP also recommends that the oncologic care of a
child or adolescent with cancer be coordinated by a pediatric hematologist/
oncologist who is board-certified or board-eligible in the subspecialty of
pediatric hematology and oncology by the American Board of Pediatrics.
By 2002, 1,740 pediatric hematology/oncology physician specialists had
been board certified (*http://www.abp.org/STATS/numdips.htm*, accessed
March 25, 2003) (roughly 80 percent of these physicians were in practice).
The AAP also recognizes many other professionals as essential members of
the cancer care health care team, including nurses, social workers, and
psychologists. In 2003, there were an estimated 2,000 active members of
the Association of Pediatric Oncology Nurses (APON) (Louise S. Miller,
Executive Director, APON, personal communication to Maria Hewitt,
March 24, 2003) and roughly 250 members of the Association of Pediatric

TABLE 5.1 Continued

Characteristic	Ambulatory Visits		Hospital Discharges	
	Annual population estimate[a]	% (se)	Annual population estimate[a]	% (se)
Main payment source				
Private	373,300	61.7 (3.7)	12,300	59.7 (2.0)
Medicaid	38,800	6.4 (1.8)	6,300	30.6 (1.6)
Uninsured	39,800	6.6 (1.9)	550	2.7 (0.5)
Other/unknown[c]	153,700	25.3 (3.4)	1,430	6.9 (1.7)
Site of care[d]				
Specialty setting	278,900	46.1 (3.8)	12,040	58.5 (7.2)
Non-specialty setting	326,700	53.9 (3.8)	8,530	41.4 (7.3)

NOTE: n = sample size; % = percent distribution; se = standard error.

[a]Annual estimates for the number of ambulatory care visits are based on a 5-year average (1995-1999). A total of 528 cases from NAMCS and NHAMCS were weighted to obtain population estimates. A total of 4,430 cases from HCUP, 1997, were weighted to obtain an annual estimate for hospital care. Numbers may not add to total because of rounding errors.

[b]Values are missing for 22.6% of cases for hospital discharges.

[c]An estimated 7% of the "other/unknown" category are insured by Medicare. Other sources of insurance include the military.

[d]For ambulatory care, specialty setting is a hospital outpatient department, and non specialty setting is a physician's office. For hospital care, a specialty setting is an urban teaching hospital and non-specialty setting is a rural or urban non teaching hospital.

SOURCES: National Ambulatory Medical Care Survey (NAMCS) and National Hospital Ambulatory Medical Care Survey (NHAMCS), 1995-1999; Healthcare Cost and Utilization Project (HCUP), 1997; special tabulations, NCPB staff.

Oncology Social Workers (APOSW) (June McAtee, APOSW Membership Chair, personal communication to Maria Hewitt, March 21, 2003).

Pediatric cancer care is usually delivered through academic centers involved in research (Wittes, 2003). Roughly 50 to 60 percent of all children and adolescents newly diagnosed with cancer in the United States are enrolled on clinical trials (Murphy, 2002; Shochat et al., 2001). This is quite remarkable, given that fewer than 5 percent of adults newly diagnosed with cancer are enrolled in trials. Clinical trials establish standards for an appropriate diagnostic workup, review of pathology, surgical approach, radiotherapy, and chemotherapy administration, as well as therapeutic efficacy and toxicity. Peer-reviewed treatment plans have provided standards of care that have diffused into community practice and benefited all patients, whether participating in clinical trials or not (Simone and Lyons, 1998) (clinical trials are discussed further in Chapter 8).

Beginning in the 1960s, evaluations of cancer treatment were organized through major pediatric centers (e.g., St Jude Children's Research Hospital, Dana Farber Cancer Institute) and national cooperative groups. The major pediatric clinical trials groups based in North America—the Children's Cancer Group (CCG), the Pediatric Oncology Group (POG), the Intergroup Rhabdomyosarcoma Study Group (IRS) and the National Wilms' Tumor Study Group (NWTSG)—merged in 2001 to form a single, nationwide group, the Children's Oncology Group (COG). The Children's Oncology Group is a National Cancer Institute-supported clinical trials cooperative group devoted exclusively to childhood and adolescent cancer research (See Chapter 8 for a discussion of COG-sponsored research). It develops and coordinates cancer clinical trials conducted within its 235 member institutions, which include cancer centers of all major universities and teaching hospitals throughout the United States and Canada, as well as sites in Europe and Australia (*http://www.nccf.org/COG/index.asp*, accessed March 15, 2003). Member institutions also conduct research that is independent of COG. The location of the 213 participating U.S. institutions is shown in Figure 5.1. Three states—Montana, Wyoming, and Alaska—do not have a COG-affiliated institution and geographic access to these institutions is limited in certain areas of the West and Midwest. Despite the geographic dispersion of specialized centers, as many as 94 percent of pediatric cancer cases (under age 15) diagnosed from 1989 to 1991 were seen at an institution that was a member of the cooperative clinical trials groups (i.e., POG or CCG) (Ross et al., 1993, 1996).

Follow-Up Care

Despite the growth in the population of childhood cancer survivors, no established guidelines outline appropriate components of follow-up care or provide models of how to deliver such care. The AAP recommends that centers providing care for children and adolescents with cancer have a "mechanism for ensuring long-term follow-up of successfully treated patients, either at the original treatment center, or by a specialist who is familiar with the potential adverse effects of treatment for childhood cancer" (American Academy of Pediatrics, 1997). Some professional organizations and advocacy groups have called for assurance of specialized long-term follow-up care for survivors of childhood cancer (Alliance for Childhood Cancer, 2002; Arceci et al., 1998). Having an on-site, long term follow-up service for survivors of pediatric cancer is a requirement for COG membership. The COG membership criteria state that the "outpa-

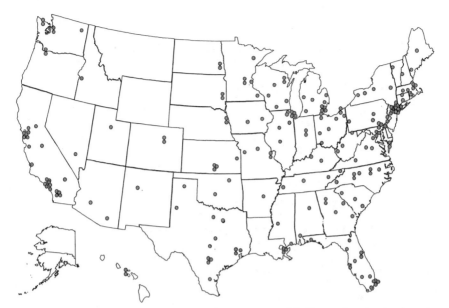

FIGURE 5.1 Map of Children's Oncology Group (COG) member institutions in the United States.
SOURCE: COG, Public Presentation Graphic, 2002.

tient clinic should ensure the long-term follow-up of successfully treated patients and those with lifelong chronic disorders" (Children's Oncology Group, 2001). The COG membership requirements are drawn from the general criteria and guidelines for pediatric cancer centers established by the Section on Hematology/Oncology of the American Academy of Pediatrics and the American Society of Pediatric Hematology/Oncology (Children's Oncology Group, 2001) (Box 5.1, sections pertaining to follow-up care are underlined).

Although many late effects of childhood cancer have been recognized, there is no clear agreement on what constitutes appropriate care. Defining the specific components of long-term services that are needed is difficult because of the variable nature of long-term outcomes associated with childhood cancer. The focus of long-term follow-up of survivors of childhood cancer should be on conditions for which effective clinical interventions are available that improve survival and/or quality of life. There are many areas for which the evidence regarding the effectiveness of follow-up care is incomplete, and for which additional research is needed. There are, however, examples of follow-up care falling into the area of prevention and psychosocial support that are supported by principles of public health and compassionate care:

Box 5.1
Requirements for Institutional Membership,
Children's Oncology Group

Required On-Site Personnel

1. Pediatric hematologist/oncologist (Board certified/eligible or equivalent)
2. Pathologist(s) (Board certified)
3. Nurses with additional training in the management of children and adolescents with cancer and blood disorders, and documented in-house training in chemotherapy administration
4. Clinical research associates trained in data management support of cooperative research
5. Respiratory therapists with expertise in pediatrics
6. Anesthesiologist with expertise in the management of children
7. Radiologist with expertise in the management of children
8. Pharmacist with expertise in chemotherapy
9. Social worker with additional training in the management of children and adolescents with cancer and blood disorders

Required On-Site Services

1. Pediatric unit
2. Intensive care unit with the ability to treat critically ill children
3. Outpatient clinic for the acute and chronic care and treatment of children and adolescents with cancer
4. Computed axial tomography
5. Ultrasonography
6. Pharmacy with capability of storage, accurate preparation, dispensing, and accounting for investigational drugs, and other antineoplastics
7. Anatomic pathology services necessary for the immediate handling of specimens and 24-hour laboratory services necessary for the care of critically ill children
8. Capabilities to provide appropriate isolation for patients with severe immunosuppression
9. Expertise available to determine the need to deliver and monitor total parenteral nutrition for critically and chronically ill children and adolescents

• Educating and counseling survivors regarding the specific risks to which they are susceptible and guidance on self-monitoring for signs of late effects.

• Applying preventive approaches known to be effective for the general population, including encouragement of abstinence from tobacco, limited exposure to alcohol, sun protection, physical activity, maintenance of a healthy weight, consumption of fruits and vegetables. At a minimum, the surveillance techniques for detecting cancer in the general population should

10. Pain management and sedation guidelines
11. *Long term follow-up services for survivors of pediatric cancer*
12. Data collection and transfer systems to support clinical trials programs

Personnel and Services That Must Be Available and Readily Accessible

Personnel

• Surgeons with expertise in the management of children: Surgeon for general surgical management (Board certified/eligible); orthopedic surgeons; urologic surgeons; neurosurgeons, plastic surgeon
• Pathologists (Board certified with special training and/or certification in 1) pediatric pathology; 2) hematopathology; 3) neuropathology
• Medical specialists/specialties: Ophthalmologist; otolaryngologist; radiation oncologists; nuclear medicine physician; pulmonology; cardiology; gastroenterology; neurology; infectious disease; endocrinology; nephrology; psychiatry
• Non-physician providers: Nutritionist(s); physical therapist(s); pediatric psychologist(s); occupational therapist(s); childlife specialist; dentistry

Services

• Diagnostic imaging and radiation oncology equipment (e.g., rotational linear accelerator)
• Clinical laboratories with expertise in the assessment and diagnosis of pediatric hematologic/oncologic disorders (Clinical Laboratory Improvement Act [CLIA] approved)
• Services for dialysis of children and adolescents
• Rehabilitation

In addition to these requirements, Comprehensive Pediatric Hematology/Oncology Programs should have regularly scheduled multidisciplinary tumor boards as well as case conferences designed to discuss children and adolescents with serious hematologic problems. *The outpatient clinic should ensure the long-term follow-up of successfully treated patients and those with lifelong chronic disorders.*

SOURCE: COG, Institutional Membership Application Procedures, 1/14/01.

be performed as recommended (e.g., screening for cancers of the breast, cervix, and colorectum).

• Providing psychosocial support services to survivors and their families.
• Providing reproductive and sexuality counseling.
• Providing genetic counseling for individuals with a hereditary cancer and their family members.

TABLE 5.2 Suggested Evaluation for Suspected Late Effects

Late effect[a]	Screening test	Recommendations if screening results abnormal
Short stature	Growth curve	Bone age, growth hormone tests
	Sitting height	Thyroid function tests[a]
	Parental heights	Endocrinologist consultation
Obesity or weight loss	Growth curve	Thyroid function tests[a]
	Diet history	Nutritionist, endocrinologist consultation
Scoliosis	Physical examination	Spine radiography; evaluate again during adolescent growth spurt
		Orthopedist consultation
Bone asymmetries (hypoplasia, atrophy)	Bone lengths, circumference	Orthopedist consultation; bone radiography; plastic surgeon consultation
Avascular necrosis or osteoporosis	History of pain, fractures	Bone scan
	Bone radiography	Serum estradiol level; Ca, P
		Orthopedist consultation; physical therapist consultation
Soft tissue hypoplasia, contractures, edema	Physical examination	Plastic surgeon consultation
Dental abnormalities	Physical examination	Dentist, oral surgeon consultation
Learning disabilities	Communication with school, family; psychological testing	CT or MRI scan of head; special education classes
Leukoencephalopathy	CT or MRI (See also Learning Disabilities, above)	Cerebrospinal fluid basic myelin protein; neurologist consultation
Neuropathy	Physical examination	Neurologist consultation
Hearing loss	Audiogram	Otorhinolaryngologist consultation; audiologist consultation
Infertility	History (primary versus secondary dysfunction)	Endocrinologist consultation
	Gonadal function testing[b]	Obstetrician or gynecologist consultation
Thyroid dysfunction	Thyroid function testing[a]	Endocrinologist consultation
Cardiomyopathy or pericarditis	Electrocardiogram; echocardiogram; radio-nuclide angiography	Cardiologist consultation
Vasoocclusive disease	Angiography; Doppler pulses	Vascular surgeon
Pneumonitis or pulmonary fibrosis	Chest radiography	Lung biopsy
	Pulmonary function tests	Pulmonologist consultation

TABLE 5.2 Continued

Late effect[a]	Screening test	Recommendations if screening results abnormal
Chronic enteritis	Growth curves Nutritional assessment	Serum folate, carotene Small-bowel studies; barium enema; gastroenterologist consultation
Hepatitis or cirrhosis	Liver function tests	Liver biopsy, hepatitis screen; liver scan; gastroenterologist consultation
Nephritis, rickets (tublar defects)	Urinalysis; BUN, creatinine, serum electrolytes, CO_2, Ca, P, alkaline phosphatase; wrist radiographs	24-h creatinine clearance or glomerular filtration rate; intravenous urogram or sonogram; nephrologist consultation
Hemorrhagic cystitis	Urinalysis	Cytoscopy; urologist consultation
Thrombotic thrombocytopenic purpura	CBC/platelets, BUN, creatinine; peripheral blood smear	
Sepsis	Compliance with prophylactic antibiotics	
Second malignancy	Studies on an individual basis	Oncologist consultation

NOTE: BUN, blood urea nitrogen; CBC, complete blood cell count; CT, computed tomography; MRI, magnetic resonance imaging.

[a]Thyroid function tests include thyroxine (T_4), thyrotropin, free T_4.

[b]Gonadal function tests: Tanner staging for boys older than 14 years at the time of evaluation or girls not yet menstruating by age 12 years or if menses become irregular; follicle-stimulating hormone, luteinizing hormone, and testosterone (semen analysis) or estradiol, as appropriate.

SOURCE: Dreyer et al., 2002. Reprinted with permission.

For many other areas of concern to survivors, there is a sufficient body of evidence to support general guidance on screening and evaluating late effects of childhood cancer. Recently published recommendations are shown in Table 5.2 (Dreyer et al., 2002). More extensive practical advice to physicians on providing follow-up care for childhood cancer survivors is available (Schwartz et al., 1994) and efforts are underway by the COG Late Effects Committee to create practice guidelines for follow-up care (Bhatia, 2002). Information on childhood cancer late effects and advice on follow-up care are also available for survivors and their families (Keene et al., 2000).

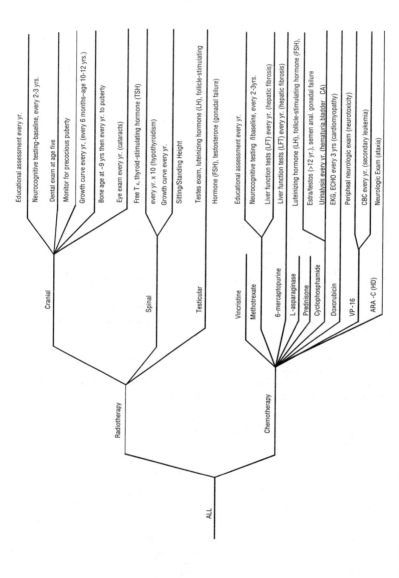

FIGURE 5.2 Follow-up of individuals treated in childhood for ALL.
SOURCE: Schwartz et al., 1994. Reprinted with permission.

While general guidance is available, there is no consensus regarding the specifics of appropriate follow-up care. Specialized long-term follow-up programs have been established, but each has tended to define its own follow-up protocols. Figure 5.2 illustrates the complexity of follow-up care showing an algorithm developed by Schwartz and her colleagues to guide follow-up care of children treated for acute lymphoblastic leukemia (ALL) (Schwartz et al., 1994). As is clear from this algorithm, practitioners providing follow-up care need to have precise information regarding the cancer diagnosis and treatments. Lacking, however, are rigorous studies to assess the cost and benefits of screening and follow-up procedures, in terms of both reduced morbidity or mortality and improved quality of life.

Assessments of late effects or the future risk of late effects may take place at the completion of primary therapy. Other assessments, including growth monitoring, could conceivably be easily integrated into routine primary care. Whether or not a distinct follow-up program is necessary to achieve appropriate levels of follow-up is uncertain and depends in large part on the level of risk faced by the cancer survivor. In the absence of specialized follow-up care, a high level of communication and support from oncology providers to the primary care provider engaged in follow-up is necessary. Despite some uncertainly regarding the details of follow-up, it is generally agreed that all survivors of childhood cancer should maintain regular contact with a health care provider who is familiar with the potential long-term health risks to which survivors are susceptible (American Academy of Pediatrics, 1997; Arceci et al., 1998; Bleyer et al., 1993; Hollen and Hobbie, 1995; Masera et al., 1996; Wallace et al., 2001).

While available guidelines support the need for a follow-up program for survivors of childhood cancer, a survey conducted in 1997 of the 219 members of the Children's Cancer Group and the Pediatric Oncology Group (groups that have since been merged into COG) indicated that only about half of them had long-term follow-up clinics (96 of 182 respondents) (Oeffinger et al., 1998). The website of the Association of Cancer Online Resources (*http://www.acor.org/ped-onc/treatment/surclinics.html*, accessed August 17, 2001) listed 28 follow-up programs that were considered comprehensive.[1] To learn more about these programs, in June and July 2001, Board staff interviewed program coordinators associated with 16 of the 28 programs listed on the website.[2]

---

[1]Comprehensive programs were those that had a dedicated time and place for the clinic, met at least twice a month, were staffed by a doctor with experience in the late effects after treatment for childhood cancer, had a nurse coordinator, provided state-of-the-art screening for individual's risk of late effects, provided referrals to appropriate specialists, and provided wellness education (*www.acor.org/ped-onc/treatment/surclinics.html*, accessed March 25, 2003).

[2] For more details of the interviews, see the background paper prepared by Eric Trabert (*www.IOM.edu/ncpb*).

All of the specialized, comprehensive, multidisciplinary follow-up programs that were contacted were located within major cancer centers and most had been developed within the past decade. The clinics function to diagnose and manage treatment-related sequelae; provide education and counseling; develop surveillance recommendations; address issues related to insurance, education, and employment; and conduct research on late effects. Pediatric nurse practitioners trained in oncology generally manage the clinics in collaboration with one or more pediatric oncologists. Additional personnel involved, usually on a referral basis, include social workers, psychologists and other specialists (e.g., cardiologists, fertility specialists, genetic counselors). Well-established programs typically assessed between 300 and 400 survivors annually, while newer programs or those serving smaller patient populations reported seeing only 50 or 60 patients each year. Most programs picked up patients after they had completed their care from their treating oncologist, generally when they were two years removed from the completion of therapy and/or three to five years from diagnosis, and disease-free. Treating oncologists generally provide follow-up for a few years following treatment to monitor for disease recurrence.

Survivors of ALL and Hodgkin's disease tended to be overrepresented in follow-up clinics, because of their relatively high risk of late effects. Another high-risk group, survivors of brain/CNS tumors, however, were not generally seen in these clinics, but were instead followed by neuro-oncology specialists. The schedule for follow-up varied depending upon factors such as patient age, initial diagnosis, and type of treatment received, but almost all programs encouraged patients to return annually for evaluation and possible diagnostic workup during the first 10 years of follow-up, or until after completion of puberty, whichever occurs later. Since puberty is a time of dramatic physical and psychological development, many late effects first present during this period and may require immediate intervention. Few follow-up programs had transition clinics that specifically targeted the needs of young adult survivors.

There are relatively few follow-up programs for survivors of adult cancer according to an informal survey of academic centers conducted for the Board (Winn, 2002). Adult survivors of childhood cancer could potentially be referred to one of these programs. Box 5.2 describes some of the programs designed to assess and manage survivorship-related concerns. A few other programs are available to address specific late effects or concerns of survivors of adult cancers (e.g., lymphedema among breast cancer survivors, sexuality, fatigue).

Although some comprehensive, specialized follow-up programs have emerged to address the concerns of cancer survivors and their families, there have been no evaluations of their effectiveness or value. As a consequence, a referral to a long-term follow-up program is often initially met by

---

Box 5.2
Characteristics of Selected Programs Serving Adult Survivors

Life After Cancer Care
University of Texas, M.D. Anderson Cancer Center

This clinic accepts individuals who have completed primary therapy and the first 1-2 years of surveillance. Staffed by an endocrinologist and nurse practitioner, the clinic emphasizes the management of endocrine dysfunction, especially premature menopause and thyroid dysfunction.

Living Well After Cancer Program
University of Pennsylvania

This program, established in 2001 with support from the Lance Armstrong Foundation, is staffed by an oncologist/epidemiologist, senior oncology nurse, social worker, and cardiology and primary care providers. Referrals are made for consultation on issues related to sexuality and genetic counseling.

Post-Treatment Resource Center
Memorial Sloan Kettering

This program is staffed by social workers and provides education, counseling, and advocacy support to cancer survivors. Lectures on survivorship, support groups, and one-on-one counseling are provided. Information and counseling on legal and discrimination issues are available.

SOURCE: Winn, 2002.

---

denial from health insurers who contend that such care is not medically necessary. Efforts to overturn these denials usually succeed in securing authorization for follow-up care, but insurers often stipulate that all lab and diagnostic tests be performed within network (Trabert, 2001). This may present logistical problems to patients who must travel extended distances to access follow-up care. In addition, reimbursement for services provided in long-term follow-up typically falls far short of compensation for the time and effort required to evaluate and manage these patients. In fact, many services garner no reimbursement for surveillance programs, including those provided by social workers, education specialists, genetic counselors, nutritionists, or dentists. Consequently, hospitals often rely on grant support or philanthropic donations to partially subsidize the costs of providing long-term follow-up care.

To what extent are survivors of childhood cancer receiving follow-up care, either at an organized clinic or through other providers? In a recent study of 635 5-year survivors of childhood cancer (members of the CCSS cohort), 44 percent stated that they had attended a clinic expressly for follow-up of their cancer (Kadan-Lottick et al., 2002). In another study of 9,434 adult survivors of childhood cancer (members of the CCSS cohort), 87 percent of survivors had had some general contact with the medical system within the previous 2 years, but only 19 percent had been seen at an oncology center or clinic, and nearly a third (30 percent) had not had a general physical examination in the past 2 years. Older age and longer time interval from cancer diagnosis were associated with lower rates of physical examination, cancer-related visits, and visits to a cancer center (Oeffinger et al., in press). Evidence suggests that once primary therapy is completed, contact with the treating institution diminishes. In the absence of formal follow-up programs, communication with patients and their families regarding the need for future care is essential. Patients and families must be able to make available to their subsequent health care providers diagnostic and treatment information needed to assess late effects.

A prerequisite to appropriate follow-up care is knowledge of what treatments were administered during primary treatment. At the conclusion of therapy, patients and their families should be provided with a summary of their treatment and informed of possible late effects and the need for follow-up care. Some evidence suggests that effective communication is not taking place. When asked in a recent study of 635 5-year survivors of childhood cancer (members of the CCSS cohort) if past therapies could cause a serious health problem with the passage of time, 35 percent responded affirmatively; 46 responded negatively; and 19 percent did not know (Kadan-Lottick et al., 2002). Only 15 percent reported that they had ever received a written statement of their disease diagnoses and treatments to keep as a reference in the future. This is consistent with preliminary results of a Robert Wood Johnson study of barriers to care among childhood cancer survivors where only 19 percent of 441 5-year survivors reported that they had been given a written summary of their treatment and could easily find it (Kevin Oeffinger, personal communication to Maria Hewitt, January 8, 2002). Many survivors and families have anecdotally reported that they were not informed of late effects or of the need for follow-up (Keene, 2002).

A sizable proportion of childhood cancer survivors lack specific knowledge of their prior diagnosis and treatment, which is information necessary to plan for future care. In the recent study of Kadan-Lottick and colleagues, 72 percent of 5-year cancer survivors could accurately identify their diagnosis. The accuracy of reporting their treatment history varied by type of treatment; accurate recall occurred among 94 percent of those who had had chemotherapy, 89 percent for radiation, and 93 percent for splenectomy.

Among those who received radiotherapy, 70 percent recalled the site of radiotherapy (Kadan-Lottick et al., 2002).

A "Cancer Patient's Treatment Record" has been developed so that survivors can print it out and request information from their treating institution (*http://patientcenters.com/survivors/*, last accessed March 15, 2003). As systems of care move toward uniform electronic medical records, individuals might be issued a "smartcard" or other electronic record of their medical history and treatment.   Ideally, at the conclusion of their treatments, cancer survivors would have information about their cancer and its treatment and an individualized plan for follow-up and guidance on preventive health practices.

Long-Term Care Needs of Children with Chronic Illness and Disability

Long-term care services may be needed by survivors of childhood cancer who have late effects that lead to functional limitations and disability. These survivors are not alone in their need for planned and coordinated follow-up care. In some cases, the clinical, psychological, educational, and other supportive interventions needed by child and adult survivors of HIV/AIDS, brain injury, hemophilia, and other conditions may also be appropriate for childhood cancer survivors. Children with special health care needs are those "who have, or are at increased risk for, chronic physical, developmental, behavioral, or emotional conditions and who also require health and related services of a type or amount beyond that required by children generally" according to the U.S. Department of Health and Human Services, Health Resources and Services Administration's Maternal and Child Health Bureau (*www.mchb.hrsa.gov*, last accessed on March 15, 2003). Figure 5.3 shows estimates made by Newacheck and colleagues of the percentage of children in the United States with chronic physical conditions, children with special health care needs (excluding at-risk children), and disability (e.g., limitations in the activities of daily living) (Newacheck et al., 1998). Nearly one in five (18 percent) of U.S. children under age 18 (13 million children) has special health care needs, excluding those at-risk children (Newacheck et al., 1998). The estimated 95,000 children and adolescents with a history of cancer would be counted among this group if they experienced late effects of treatment or if they required follow-up care or surveillance beyond that expected within the context of routine pediatric care. The additional 175,000 adult survivors of childhood cancer would require a similar designation among adults.

It may well be the case that there are common services needed by the relatively large, heterogeneous group of children with chronic conditions, special needs, and disabilities. If so, there may be opportunities to reach a large group of individuals and families who have common needs with

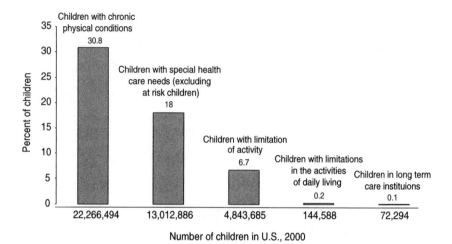

FIGURE 5.3 Prevalence of chronic conditions, special needs, and disability among children under age 18.
SOURCE: Adapted from Newacheck et al., 1998.

services delivered outside of a disease-specific context. There is some rationale for this insofar as therapeutic goals for chronically ill children and their families are different from those of children with acute illness. Some common goals include integration into community life, enhancing child and family responsibility for self-care, and optimal social and educational development (Perrin and Starr, 1993). An array of health and family support services are often needed to meet these therapeutic goals, and coordination of services becomes central to the provision of care. Care coordination is often complicated because there is no single entry point to multiple systems of care, and complex criteria determine the availability of funding and services among public and private payers of care (Ziring et al., 1999). Families themselves usually assume most of the care coordination responsibilities for children with cancer, but health care providers can play a vital role in concert with families. The concept of a "medical home" has been developed to ensure that medical care is accessible, continuous, comprehensive, family centered, coordinated, compassionate, and culturally effective (American Academy of Pediatrics, 2002a). The medical home is a source of ongoing community-based routine health care whereby providers and families work as partners to meet the needs of children and family (*http://www.mchb.hrsa.gov/programs/specialneeds/measuresuccess.htm*, accessed March 15, 2003). The medical home assists in the early identification of special health care needs; provides ongoing primary care; and coordinates with a broad range of other specialty, ancillary, and related services. The need of a medical home is especially important for children with special health care needs and the U.S. Department of Health and Human Services Healthy People 2010 goals and objectives state that "all children with special health care needs will receive regular ongoing comprehensive care within a medical home" (*http://www.mchb.hrsa.gov/programs/specialneeds/measuresuccess.htm*, accessed March 15, 2003).

Acute care insurance policies often cover a limited number of supportive services such as home care, physical therapy, or occupational therapy services following an acute episode of illness, but generally this coverage does not extend beyond certain time limits. Supportive services needed to maintain function after an acute episode has resolved are usually excluded from health insurance policies. A number of public and private programs are available to fill in the gaps, but parents often complain of a patchwork of available services that are often hard to learn about and access.

Several federal programs help to finance or deliver home- and community-based long-term supportive services. The Supplemental Security Income (SSI) program of the Social Security Administration (SSA), for example, offers cash assistance to poor families whose children meet SSA's medical disability eligibility criteria. Once determined eligible for SSI, a child becomes eligible for Medicaid, an important source of acute and long-term care services. The Medicare program covers Americans living with disabilities and those with end-stage renal disease (Medicaid, SSI, and Medicare programs are reviewed in Chapter 7). Long-term care services are also often available through federally supported, state-run Children with Special Health Care Needs programs (these Title V programs are described in Chapter 7). The largest federal program serving children with disabilities is delivered through the public school system. Young children with disabilities are eligible for the "Part H" program, and older children can benefit from special education and "related services" that can include supportive long-term care services such as occupational and physical therapy (educational programs are described in Chapter 6).

Selected private organizations involved in advocacy and the provision of supportive services for families of children with cancer are described in Box 5.3. These programs provide information, peer support, special services such as camping programs, and opportunities for advocacy.

Alternate Models of Delivery of Follow-Up Care

While there is consensus that the primary treatment of childhood cancer requires specialized care, and that a plan for follow-up should be in place for all survivors of childhood cancer, it is unclear whether oncology-based specialized follow-up care is the only appropriate model of care to meet the long-terms needs of survivors of childhood cancer. Are oncology-

Box 5.3
Services for Children with Cancer and Their Families Offered by Selected Voluntary Organizations

SUPPORT GROUPS/PROGRAMS

• **Candlelighters Childhood Cancer Foundation Regional Organizations** located in all U.S. states provide speakers, parent meetings, support groups and other services (*http://candlelighters.org/support.stm*).

• **The Children's Brain Tumor Foundation** assists in the development of regional and local support groups, internet conferences, and other resources for pediatric brain tumor patients and their families.

• **National Children's Cancer Society** sponsors nationwide programs dedicated to improving the lives of children with cancer. The *Pediatric Oncology Program* promotes advocacy, emotional support, and financial assistance for families who have a child with cancer. The *Letting Kids Be Kids Program* provides psychosocial support for children with cancer by fostering supportive environments, offering entertaining and educational activities, and promoting a sense of normalcy in the lives of children with cancer (*http://www.children-cancer.com*).

• **Ulman Cancer Fund for Young Adults** provides support, education, and resources for young adults, their families and friends, affected by cancer (*www.ulmanfund.org*).

• **American Cancer Society (ACS)** offers a program that helps teenage cancer patients cope with the effects of cancer treatment called *Look Good...Feel Better for Teens* (*http://www.cancer.org/eprise/main/docroot/SHR/content/SHR_2.1_x_Look_Good_Feel_Better_for_Teens?sitearea=SHR*).

based follow-up programs always advisable? Are alternative models of care needed that are based in primary care? In part, the answer to these questions depends on an understanding of the unique characteristics of the pediatric cancer care system and the distinct follow-up care needs among survivors of childhood cancer.

An argument for specialized follow-up programs within cancer centers can be made on the basis of the multidiciplinary expertise represented in such institutions and their familiarity with late effects. It is likely that persistent concerns regarding cancer recurrence can best be addressed in these settings. The fact that the majority of children treated for cancer are cared for in specialized centers also points to the advantage of continuity should follow-up care be assumed by the institutions initially treating the cancer. The primary treating oncologist is already providing a considerable amount of follow-up care. Oncologists and their colleagues typically fol-

ONLINE SUPPORT

• **Association of Cancer Online Resources** organizes a number of list-servs and chat groups, online communities, and peer support groups (e.g., BMT-TALK, PED-ONC) (*http://www.acor.org/mailing.html*).
• **Planet Cancer** is a community of young adults with cancer that share online support, insights, and information; it also provides a clearinghouse of informal regional gatherings for support and networking (*http://www.planetcancer.org*).
• **Starbright World** is a peer-support project for children with cancer and other seriously ill children sponsored by the Starbright Foundation. It is available through 95 hospitals throughout the U.S. and provides a private computer network through which chronically or seriously ill children and teens from across the United States and Canada can interact (*http://www.starbright.org*).
• **Cancer Kids** sponsors a message board for kids to communicate about their cancer (*http://www.cancerkids.org*).
• **OncoChat** is an online support community for people whose lives have been affected by cancer (*http://www.oncochat.org*).

CAMPS

Several organizations provide camping opportunities for children with cancer.
• Happiness Is Camping (*http://www.happinessiscamping.org/about/htm*)
• Hole in the Wall Gang (*http://www.holeinthewallgang.org*)
• Camp Make-A-Dream (*http://www.campdream.org*)
• Camp Good Days and Special Times (*http://www.campgooddays.org/programs.html*)
• Camp Cancer (a virtual camp) for kids with Cancer (*http://netpressence.com/camp-cancer/*)
• Children's Oncology Camping Association International (C.O.C.A.) represents 65 member camps and provides an online directory of all C.O.C.A. camps (*http://www.coca-intl.org/information.html*).

low their patients for 2 to 3 years after the conclusion of treatment. Having pediatric oncologists provide longer-term follow-up care could effectively familiarize these providers with late effects and provide them with insights as to how best modify initial treatments to minimize adverse late sequelae.

When follow-up care is provided at a cancer center, is it necessary to have a separate clinic apart from the one where children come to be treated for their cancer? Specialized clinics were, in fact, first developed to address the limitations of follow-up within the oncology outpatient clinic. Typically, clinicians in such clinics would try to evaluate the medical and psychosocial needs of survivors during the brief time usually allotted for acute care visits. Consequently, follow-up was limited to checking for symptoms of disease recurrence or second malignant neoplasms at the expense of treating the complete physical and psychological needs of survivors. The inadequacy of this approach led some to instead develop nurse-led, multidisciplinary clinics with a more holistic approach as described earlier (Hobbie and Hollen, 1993). Such programs also facilitate the collection of extensive data for medical research.

Another reason why separate follow-up clinics were developed was in response to cancer survivors' reluctance to return to the clinic where they received treatment. A return to the clinic, amidst patients who are receiving active therapy, can stir up unpleasant and sometimes painful memories. Some programs, however, favor holding follow-up in the acute care setting because it facilitates the establishment of mentoring programs between survivors and newly diagnosed patients.

Since late effects may not emerge until several years after treatment is completed, it is important to maintain active follow-up of childhood cancer survivors as they transition through adolescence and into adulthood (MacLean et al., 1996; Oeffinger et al., 1998). A distinct disadvantage of having follow-up clinics in pediatric settings is the difficulty of involving clinicians who understand how therapy given during childhood manifests as health problems in adults. Some speculate that many adolescent and young adult survivors are lost to follow-up simply because they do not want to receive care in a pediatric institution, perhaps feeling that they have outgrown the type of care normally provided in this setting. The American Academy of Pediatrics issued a policy statement in 1996 and a consensus statement in 2002 to guide pediatricians as they assist adolescents with special health care needs to positively adapt within an adult-focused system of health care (American Academy of Pediatrics, 1996; 2002).[3]

Potential advantages to having follow-up take place in the primary care setting include gaining a sense of a return to normalcy; getting care within the context of total health needs and with one's familiar practitioner; and avoidance of trips to a cancer center that may be far from home. Importantly, a child's pediatrician can play a pivotal role as a support to, and community advocate for, the child and family (Pizzo, 1990). The schedule of visits for preventive pediatric health care recommended by the American Academy of Pediatrics is shown in Box 5.4 (*http://www.aap.org/policy/re9939.html*, accessed March 15, 2003). Some cancer-related follow-up care might be provided during routinely scheduled visits. Other follow-up care might involve additional visits or referrals to other providers.

Since many late effects will not show up immediately after treatment, the need for follow-up care may first be recognized during adulthood when individuals have established ties to adult primary care providers. Survivors may wish to remain under the care of their adult primary care provider for the management of any late effects.

---

[3]The American Academy of Pediatrics consensus statement is summarized in chapter 9.

Potential disadvantages to having follow-up take place in the primary care setting could include the primary care provider lacking knowledge about late effects and their management, and a lack of expertise in certain aspects of the physical exam important in detecting cancer recurrence. Some of these disadvantages can be overcome with appropriate levels of communication between oncology and primary care providers and with the provision of education and training opportunities.

With improved survival among children who have had cancer, primary care physicians will increasingly become involved in their long-term follow-up. But despite the growing numbers of survivors, visits made by such children and young adults will be rare events for the typical pediatrician, family practitioner, or internist. Innovative methods are needed to alert these providers to the unique needs of these patients. There have been recent calls for research on the organization of care for children with disabilities, and in particular, on ways to enhance communication and collaboration between primary and subspecialty care providers (Perrin, 2002).

Defining Quality Survivorship Care

Irrespective of who provides survivorship care or where it is provided, an ideal system of survivorship care would:

- provide a range of direct services to survivors to identify, prevent, treat, and ameliorate late effects,
- bridge the realms of primary and specialty health care with education and outreach,
- coordinate medical care with educational and occupational services, and
- conduct research to better understand late effects and their prevention.

These functions of an ideal follow-up system of care for survivors of childhood cancer are described in Box 5.5. Implicit in the "ideal" is the goal to improve outcomes of survivors of childhood cancer. The system described includes evaluations of effectiveness of interventions to ameliorate late effects and measure the prevalence of late effects. These two activities would likely yield results that would inform the success of the proposed follow-up system.

There are different models of care through which appropriate follow-up care might be attained (Harvey et al., 1999; Hollen and Hobbie, 1995; Oeffinger, 2002; Oeffinger et al., 1998; Wallace et al., 2001). The one described most frequently in the literature relies on the development of specialized long-term follow-up clinics, usually at a cancer center.

Box 5.4 Recommendations for Preventive Pediatric Health Care (RE9939)

Committee on Practice and Ambulatory Medicine

Each child and family is unique; therefore, **these Recommendations for Preventive Pediatric Health Care** are designed for the care of children who are receiving competent parenting, have no manifestations of any important health problems,

				INFANCY[4]
AGE[5]	PRENATAL[1]	NEWBORN[2]	2-4d[3]	By 1mo
HISTORY				
Initial/Interval	•	•	•	•
MEASUREMENTS				
Height and Weight		•	•	•
Head Circumference		•	•	•
Blood Pressure				
SENSORY SCREENING				
Vision		S	S	S
Hearing		O[7]	S	S
DEVELOPMENTAL/ BEHAVIORAL ASSESMENT[8]		•	•	•
PHYSICAL EXAMINATION[9]		•	•	•
PROCEDURES-GENERAL[10]				
Hereditary/Metabolic Screening[11]		··	•	→
Immunization[12]		•	•	•
Hematocrit or Hemoglobin[13]				
Urinalysis				
PROCEDURES-PATIENTS AT RISK				
Lead Screening[16]				
Tuberculin Test[17]				
Cholesterol Screening[18]				
STD Screening[19]				
Pelvic Exam[20]				
ANTICIPATORY GUIDANCE[21]	•	•	•	•
Injury Prevention[22]	•	•	•	•
Violence Prevention[23]	•	•	•	•
Sleep Positioning Counseling[24]	•	•	•	•
Nutrition Counseling[25]	•	•	•	•
DENTAL REFERRAL[26]				

and are growing and developing in satisfactory fashion. **Additional visits may become necessary** if circumstances suggest variations from normal. These guidelines represent a consensus by the Committee on Practice and Ambulatory Medicine in consultation with national committees and sections of the American Academy of Pediatrics. The Committee emphasize the great importance of **continuity of care** in comprehensive health supervision and the need to avoid **fragmentation of care.**

EARLY CHILDHOOD[4]

2mo	4mo	6mo	9mo	12mo	15mo	18mo	24mo	3y	4y
•	•	•	•	•	•	•	•	•	•
•	•	•	•	•	•	•	•	•	•
•	•	•	•	•	•	•	•		
								•	•
S	S	S	S	S	S	S	S	O[6]	O
S	S	S	S	S	S	S	S	S	O
•	•	•	•	•	•	•	•	•	•
•	•	•	•	•	•	•	•	•	•
•	•	•	•	•	•	•	•	★	•
			•	→	★	★	★	★	★
		★	→				★		
			★	★	★	★	★	★	★
							★	★	★
•	•	•	•	•	•	•	•	•	•
•	•	•	•	•	•	•	•	•	•
•	•	•	•	•	•	•	•	•	•
•	•	•							
•	•	•	•	•	•	•	•	•	•
			←	←	←	←	•		

continued on next page

Box 5.4 Recommendations for
Preventive Pediatric Health Care (RE9939) *continued*

AGE[5]	MIDDLE CHILDHOOD[4]					
	5y	6y	8y	10y	11y	12y
HISTORY						
Initial/Interval	•	•	•	•	•	•
MEASUREMENTS						
Height and Weight	•	•	•	•	•	•
Head Circumference						
Blood Pressure	•	•	•	•	•	•
SENSORY SCREENING						
Vision	O	O	O	O	S	O
Hearing	O	O	O	O	S	O
DEVELOPMENTAL/						
BEHAVIORAL ASSESMENT[8]	•	•	•	•	•	•
PHYSICAL EXAMINATION[9]	•	•	•	•	•	•
PROCEDURES-GENERAL[10]						
Hereditary/Metabolic Screening[11]						
Immunization[12]	•	•	•	•	•	•
Hematocrit or Hemoglobin[13]	*				←	←
Urinalysis	•				←	←
PROCEDURES-PATIENTS AT RISK						
Lead Screening[16]						
Tuberculin Test[17]		*	*	*	*	*
Cholesterol Screening[18]		*	*	*	*	*
STD Screening[19]					*	*
Pelvic Exam[20]					*	*
ANTICIPATORY GUIDANCE[21]	•	•	•	•	•	•
Injury Prevention[22]	•	•	•	•	•	•
Violence Prevention[23]	•	•	•	•	•	•
Sleep Positioning Counseling[24]						
Nutrition Counseling[25]	•	•	•	•	•	•
DENTAL REFERRAL[26]						

ADOLESCENCE[4]

13y	14y	15y	16y	17y	18y	19y	20y	21y
•	•	•	•	•	•	•	•	•
•	•	•	•	•	•	•	•	•
•	•	•	•	•	•	•	•	•
S	S	O	S	S	O	S	S	S
S	S	O	S	S	O	S	S	S
•	•	•	•	•	•	•	•	•
•	•	•	•	•	•	•	•	•
•	•	•	•	•	•	•	•	•
•14	→	→	→	→	→	→	→	→
←	←	→	•15	→	→	→	→	→
★	★	★	★	★	★	★	★	★
★	★	★	★	★	★	★	★	★
★	★	★	★	★	★	★	★	★
★	★	★	★	★	★	★20	★	★
•	•	•	•	•	•	•	•	•
•	•	•	•	•	•	•	•	•
•	•	•	•	•	•	•	•	•
•	•	•	•	•	•	•	•	•

continued on next page

**Box 5.4 Recommendations for
Preventive Pediatric Health Care (RE9939)** *continued*

1. A prenatal visit is recommended for parents who are at risk, for first-time parents, and for those who request a conference. The prenatal visit should include anticipatory guidance, pertinent medical history, and a discussion of benefits of breastfeeding and

2. Planned method of feeding per AAP statement "The Prenatal Visit" (1996).

3. Every infant should have a newborn evaluation after birth. Breastfeeding should be encouraged and instruction and support offered. Every breast feeding infant should have an evaluation 48-72 hours after discharge from the hospital to include weight, formal breast feeding evaluation, encouragement, and instruction as recommended in the AAP statement "Breast Feeding and the Use of Human Milk" (1997).

4. For newborns discharged in less than 48 hours after delivery per AAP statement "Hospital Stay for Healthy Term Newborns" (1995).

5. Developmental, psychosocial, and chronic disease issues for children and adolescents may require frequent counseling and treatment visits separate from preventive care visits.

6. If a child comes under care for the first time at any point on the schedule, or if any items are not accomplished at the suggested age, the schedule should be brought up to date at the earliest possible time.

7. If the patient is uncooperative, rescreen within 6 months.

8. All newborns should be screened per AAP Task Force on Newborn and Infant Hearing statement, "Newborn and Infant Hearing Loss: Detection and Intervention" (Erenberg et al., 1999).

9. By history and appropriate physical examination: if suspicious, by specific objective developmental testing. Parenting skills should be fostered at every visit.

10. At each visit, a complete physical examination is essential, with infant totally unclothed, older child undressed and suitably draped.

11. These may be modified, depending upon entry point into schedule and individual need.

12. Metabolic screening (e.g., thyroid, hemoglobinopathies, PKU, galactosemia) should be done according to state law.

13. Schedule(s) per Committee on Infectious Diseases, published annually in the January edition of *Pediatrics*. Every visit should be an opportunity to update and complete a child's immunizations.

14. See AAP *Pediatric Nutrition Handbook* (1998) for a discussion of universal and selective screening options. Consider earlier screening for high-risk infants (e.g., premature infants and low birth weight infants). See also "Recommendations to Prevent and Control Iron Deficiency in the United States." *MMWR.* 1998;47 (RR-3):1-29.

15. All menstruating adolescents should be screened annually.

16. Conduct dipstick urinalysis for leukocytes annually for sexually active male and female adolescents.

17. For children at risk of lead exposure consult the AAP statement "Screening for Elevated Blood Levels" (1998). Additionally, screening should be done in accordance with state law where applicable.

18. TB testing per recommendations of the Committee on Infectious Diseases, published in the current edition of *Red Book: Report of the Committee on Infectious Diseases*. Testing should be done upon recognition of high-risk factors.

19. Cholesterol screening for high-risk patients per AAP statement "Cholesterol in Childhood" (1998). If family history cannot be ascertained and other risk factors are present, screening should be at the discretion of the physician.

20. All sexually active patients should be screened for sexually transmitted diseases (STDs).

21. All sexually active females should have a pelvic examination. A pelvic examination and routine Pap smear should be offered as part of preventive health maintenance between the ages of 18 and 21 years.

22. Age-appropriate discussion and counseling should be an integral part of each visit for care per the AAP *Guidelines for Health Supervision III* (1998).

23. From birth to age 12, refer to the AAP injury prevention program (TIPP®) as described in *A Guide to Safety Counseling in Office Practice* (1994).

24. Violence prevention and management for all patients per AAP Statement "The Role of Pediatrician in Youth Violence Prevention in Clinical Practice and at the Community Level" (1999).

25. Parents and caregivers should be advised to place healthy infants on their backs when putting them to sleep. Side positioning is a reasonable alternative but carries a slightly higher risk of SIDS. Consult the AAP statement "Changing Concepts of Sudden Infant Death Syndrome: Implications for Infant Sleeping Environment and Sleep Position" (2000).

26. Age-appropriate nutrition counseling should be an integral part of each visit per the AAP *Handbook of Nutrition* (1998).

27. Earlier initial dental examinations may be appropriate for some children. Subsequent examinations as prescribed by dentist.

Key: • = to be performed   * = to be performed for patients at risk
S = subjective, by history   O = objective, by a standard testing method
← • → = the range during which a service may be provided, with the dot indicating the preferred age.

SOURCE: *www.aap.org/policy/re9939.html.*

Box 5.5
Functions of an Ideal Follow-Up System for Survivors of Childhood Cancer

Provide services

- Identify late effects (or the risk of late effects)
- Review prior disease history and treatments
- Conduct clinical examinations and tests
- Evaluate symptoms
- Develop plan for long-term surveillance
- Coordinate specialists involved in diagnosis and treatment of late effects (e.g, cardiologists, neurologists)
- Ameliorate late effects through rehabilitation services (e.g., physical therapy, occupational therapy)
- Provide psychosocial support
- Counsel regarding educational and occupational issues
- Counsel regarding disease prevention, health promotion
- Refer to clinical trial or other research initiative
- Provide care coordination/case management (including the transition from pediatric to adult care)
- Provide family-based care and education and outreach to survivors and their families in the community

Educate and train professionals

- Consult with primary care providers
- Consult with schools and educators
- Provide long-term perspective to oncology care providers
- Alert providers and researchers to new late effects
- Train primary care and oncology care providers

Conduct research

- Measure prevalence of late effects
- Identify etiology of late effects
- Evaluate effectiveness of interventions to ameliorate late effects
- Evaluate and modify treatment approaches to minimize late effects
- Develop standards of follow-up care

The Late Effects Committee of the United Kingdom Children's Cancer Study Group has recently suggested a tiered approach with postal or telephone contacts made with those at lowest risk of late effects, follow-up by a nurse or primary care doctor for those at moderate risk, and a medically supervised late effects clinic for those with high risk of late effects (Wallace et al., 2001) (Table 5.3).

TABLE 5.3 Possible Levels of Follow-Up More Than 5 Years from Completion of Treatment

Level	Treatment	Method of follow-up	Frequency	Examples of tumors
1	• Surgery alone • Low risk chemotherapy	Mail or telephone	1-2 years	• Wilms' tumor stage I or II • Langerhans cell histiocytosis (single system disease) • Germ cell tumors (surgery only)
2	• Chemotherapy • Low dose cranial irradiation (<24 Gy)	Led by nurse or primary care doctor	1-2 years	• Most patients (e.g., ALL in first remission)
3	• Radiotherapy, except low dose cranial irradiation • Megatherapy	Medically supervised late effects clinic	Annual	• Brain tumors • After bone marrow transplant • Patients with stage IV tumors (any tumor type)

SOURCE: Wallace et al., 2001.

A novel strategy for long-term follow-up has been proposed that relies extensively on distance networking through the Internet and telecommunication technologies (Oeffinger, 2002). This model would link the survivor to a nationally supported center that would be responsible for facilitating health care needs. The center would have four components: a national cancer registry, care coordinators, a repository of information, and a decision-making board. Upon diagnosis of cancer, children would be entered in the registry. Upon completion of primary therapy, the treating cancer center would provide the national center with a summary of treatment and complications. Care coordinators would develop a survivor-specific plan of action, assess health care resources in the survivor's environment, and orchestrate care with appropriate health care providers located near the survivor. The repository would include guidelines for screening and surveillance, current literature about survivor-related health care problems and needs, and patient and physician education materials. The board, including health care providers and survivors, would garner necessary resources to facilitate and enhance the process.

A comprehensive regional approach to providing follow-up care to survivors of childhood cancer has been adopted by the Canadian province of Ontario (Greenberg, 2002). A network of after-care programs is being set up by the Pediatric Oncology Group of Ontario (POGO) to extend follow-up care through adulthood. The program integrates research and health care, with a focus on clinical care, surveillance, and health promotion and disease prevention. A set of consensus algorithms and guidelines is available to providers. Figure 5.4 illustrates one of their algorithms, a strategy for providing neuropsychological testing for long-term survivors of childhood cancer.

Aftercare through the POGO program generally begins two years after completion of all therapy (or four years from diagnosis). Visits are annual for up to 10 years following diagnosis and biannual thereafter, although in some specified circumstances, visits may be made more frequently (e.g., when growth failure is being monitored). An essential component of the program is a "Passport to Health," which is a credit card sized, portable, comprehensive abbreviated summary of diagnosis, treatment, complications, potential adverse effects, hepatitis status, and other relevant information necessary for the survivor and his or her health care practitioners. In the area of health education, counseling is provided to minimize risk, written materials are provided on prevention and aftercare, and links to sources of information (e.g., books, websites) are given. A centralized database will link childhood treatment data to outcomes using standardized data collection procedures. Some sites of care will be in a pediatric setting, while others will be incorporated in internal medicine programs or adult-based cancer centers. Services to residents of remote areas will be provided by a traveling team of oncology experts. This system, while still in its development, appears to incorporate many of the ideal components outlined at the beginning of this chapter.

An interesting model of health care delivery and research outside of the area of cancer is a program of the Cystic Fibrosis Foundation (CFF) that accredits a network of more than 115 care centers across the United States.[4] CFF-accredited centers must meet criteria for personnel, facilities, services, and research (*www.cff.org/chapters_and_care_centers/*, last accessed March 15, 2003). Care is provided according to CFF clinical practice guidelines developed by an advisory group of CF experts. Consensus conferences are held to update guidelines. A central patient registry tracks the health of

---

[4]Cystic fibrosis is a genetic disease caused by a single gene defect that results in the faulty transport of salt in organs such as the lungs and the pancreas. The defective gene causes the body to produce thick, sticky mucus that blocks the ducts in these organs, disrupting their normal functions (CFF, 2002).

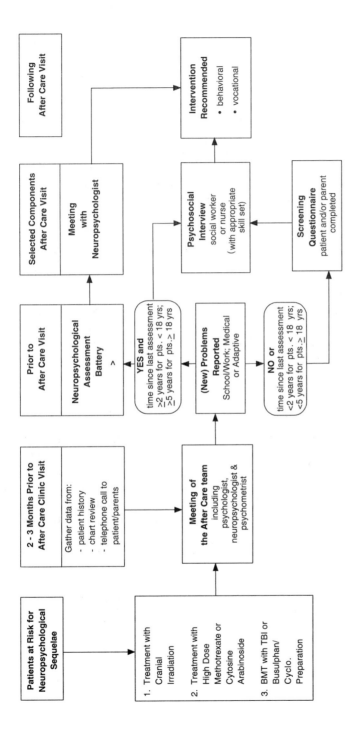

FIGURE 5.4 Neuropsychological testing for long-term survivors of childhood cancer—Pediatric Oncology Group of Ontario.
SOURCE: Greenberg, 2002.

patients enrolled in CFF clinics and analyses of these data have provided new insights into the consequences of the disease (e.g., growth and development, reproduction), treatment, and preventive health strategies (Cystic Fibrosis Foundation, 2002). The dual focus on guideline-driven standardized care and research is an attractive feature of this program and such an initiative should be considered for its applicability to survivors of childhood cancer.

To date, there have been no demonstration projects to assess alternative models of delivery and no evaluations of existing programs of follow-up care to survivors of childhood cancer. It is likely that multiple models of care will be needed to accommodate the varied circumstances and preferences of survivors and families. For some survivors, long-term follow-up clinics will serve survivors' needs best. For other survivors, primary care providers may be able to provide the most appropriate follow-up care, especially as other chronic illnesses of age develop. We do not yet know what will work best. Demonstration and research programs conducted under the discretionary grant programs of the Maternal and Child Health Block Grant Program may inform the development of delivery systems appropriate for cancer survivors. These programs have included initiatives aimed at improving care for individuals with hemophilia, sickle cell anemia, and traumatic brain injury (see a description of selected grants in Chapter 7).

Statewide Comprehensive Cancer Control

Opportunities in the United States to develop regional approaches to care for childhood cancer survivors could be facilitated by the Centers for Disease Control and Prevention (CDC) efforts to build the capacities of states—and, in turn, their local partners—to both develop and implement comprehensive cancer control plans. As part of CDC's National Comprehensive Cancer Control Program, such plans have been defined as those with an integrated and coordinated approach to reducing the incidence and the rates of morbidity and mortality from cancer through prevention, early detection, treatment, rehabilitation, and palliation (*www.cdc.gov/cancer/ncccp/index.htm*, accessed March 15, 2003).

CDC has identified a useful framework for the establishment of a state cancer control program and has provided various models for comprehensive planning and evaluation. Essential elements of a comprehensive plan include (Abed et al., 2000a; Abed et al., 2000b) the following:

- strategies and mechanisms for developing and maintaining partnerships,
- assessments and surveillance,

- infrastructure development,
- public education,
- professional education,
- policy and legislative activities, and
- evaluation and monitoring.

Phases of implementation of a comprehensive state plan include setting optimal objectives that are data-driven, determining optimal strategies that are science-driven, establishing feasible priorities given the capacity, and implementing effective strategies that are assessed by evaluations of outcomes (Abed et al., 2000a; Abed et al., 2000b). Many states have in place some of the essential elements of a comprehensive program. Nearly half of the states, for example, have cancer registries that achieve standards of completeness, timeliness, and coverage to provide accurate cancer incidence data for planning and evaluation. According to a recent CDC assessment, however, only 13 states have comprehensive state plans that are being implemented (or that are ready to be implemented), 14 states and the District of Columbia are creating a new plan (or are updating an old plan), and 23 states have no plan or one that is outdated (Figure 5.5).

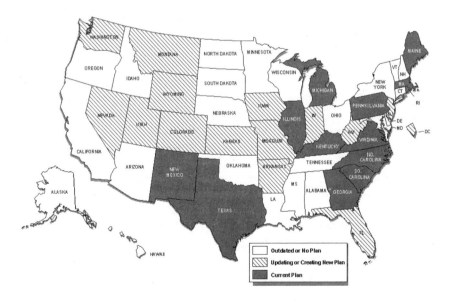

FIGURE 5.5 Comprehensive cancer control plans, 2001.
SOURCE: L. Given, CDC, Division of Cancer Prevention and Control, personal communication to Maria hewitt, July 10, 2001.

Although considerable variations in state capacities have been observed and certain barriers to implementation have been identified, it is unclear what levels and types of investment are needed to build state and local capacities and how these needs may vary across the nation. CDC's Division of Cancer Prevention and Control spends an estimated $250 million on cancer control and prevention annually, but much of the money is categorically targeted to specific activities (e.g., cancer registries), populations, or cancer sites. Since 1998, 19 states and 1 tribal organization have received grant support totalling approximately $37 million from CDC to develop and implement a comprehensive cancer control (CCC) plan. In addition, states and tribal organizations have been provided technical assistance regarding CCC plans with $1 million from the CDC (Leslie Given, Division of Cancer Prevention and Control, CDC, personal communication to Maria Hewitt, September 9, 2002). The CDC-funded states are developing a variety of programs, depending on the needs and organizational preferences of each state. The key to each program is, however, the same—fostering collaborative efforts among many sectors within the states to increase individual and organizational awareness of the state's cancer burden and to achieve objectives that will lead to future reductions in that burden (Tim Byers, University of Colorado School of Medicine, unpublished). Resources appear to be inadequate to meet the need for CCC plan development and implementation. In 2002, for example, CDC had resources to support only half of the requests for assistance from states, territories, and Indian tribes in response to its National Cancer Prevention and Control Program Announcement (Leslie Given, Division of Cancer Prevention and Control, CDC, personal communication to Maria Hewitt, IOM, August 26, 2002). The CDC estimates that $30 million per year would be needed before states would have plans developed and implementation in progress by 2005 (Leslie Given, Division of Cancer Prevention and Control, CDC, personal communication to Maria Hewitt, IOM, August 26, 2002).

A bill recently introduced in Congress, the Cancer Survivorship Research and Quality of Life Act of 2002 (HR 4963), calls for expansion of CDC comprehensive cancer programs to improve cancer survivorship. Among its provisions is support of innovative post-treatment programs, services, and demonstrations designed to support and advance cancer survivorship. Comprehensive state plans have potential, but to date, very few have addressed issues related to pediatric cancer or to survivorship issues.

SUMMARY AND CONCLUSIONS

Fifty to sixty percent of children with cancer are initially treated in specialized cancer centers, but somewhat fewer—an estimated 40-45 percent—are receiving follow-up care in specialized clinics. A disturbing finding from recent research is that the majority of cancer survivors appear to be unaware of their level of risk and need for follow-up care, and to lack the specific information regarding their disease history and treatment that would be needed by a clinician to provide appropriate care.

The need for a plan for survivorship follow-up care is widely acknowledged and general recommendations for such care are available to clinicians, survivors, and their families. An active research program is needed to address the many outstanding questions regarding the necessary components of follow-up care in the identification, prevention, and amelioration of specific late effects. Needed also are evaluations of models of care to assess which of them confer benefits in terms of preventing or ameliorating late effects and improving quality of life, and which survivors might prefer. Cancer survivors, while having some unique needs, have similarities with survivors of other chronic illness. There are likely opportunities to develop efficient systems of care to address at least some of the needs of individuals with a broad range of chronic illnesses and conditions.

REFERENCES

Abed J, Reilley B, Butler MO, Kean T, Wong F, Hohman K. 2000a. Comprehensive cancer control initiative of the Centers for Disease Control and Prevention: an example of participatory innovation diffusion. *J Public Health Manag Pract* 6(2):79-92.

Abed J, Reilley B, Butler MO, Kean T, Wong F, Hohman K. 2000b. Developing a framework for comprehensive cancer prevention and control in the United States: an initiative of the Centers for Disease Control and Prevention. *J Public Health Manag Pract* 6(2):67-78.

Alliance for Childhood Cancer. 2002. *Core Principles for Comprehensive Quality Cancer Care for Children and Adolescents.* Washington, DC: Alliance for Childhood Cancer Care.

American Academy of Pediatrics. 1996. Transition of care provided for adolescents with special health care needs. American Academy of Pediatrics Committee on Children with Disabilities and Committee on Adolescence. *Pediatrics* 98(6 Pt 1):1203-6.

American Academy of Pediatrics. 1997. Guidelines for the pediatric cancer center and role of such centers in diagnosis and treatment. American Academy of Pediatrics Section Statement Section on Hematology/Oncology. *Pediatrics* 99(1):139-41.

American Academy of Pediatrics. 2002a. The medical home. *Pediatrics* 110(1 Pt 1):184-6.

American Academy of Pediatrics. 2002b. A consensus statement on health care transitions for young adults with special health care needs. *Pediatrics* 110(6 Pt 2):1304-6.

Arceci RJ, Reaman GH, Cohen AR, Lampkin BC. 1998. Position statement for the need to define pediatric hematology/oncology programs: a model of subspecialty care for chronic childhood diseases. Health Care Policy and Public Issues Committee of the American Society of Pediatric Hematology/Oncology. *J Pediatr Hematol Oncol* 20(2):98-103.

Bhatia S. 2002. Children's Oncology Group Late Effects Committtee. *National Cancer Policy Board Meeting.* Washington, DC.

Bleyer WA, Smith RA, Green DM, DeLaat CA, Lampkin BC, Coltman CA, Brady AM, Simon M, Krischer JP, Menck HR. 1993. American Cancer Society Workshop on Adolescents and Young Adults with Cancer. Workgroup #1: Long-term care and lifetime follow-up. *Cancer* 71(7):2413.

Bloom BS, Knorr RS, Evans AE. 1985. The epidemiology of disease expenses. The costs of caring for children with cancer. *JAMA* 253(16):2393-7.

Children's Oncology Group. 2001. Requirements for Institutional Membership. Arcadia, CA: COG.

Children's Oncology Group. 2002. Public Presentation Graphic. Bethesda, MD.

Cystic Fibrosis Foundation. Patient Registry 2001 Annual Report. Bethesda, MD: 2002.

Dreyer ZE, Blatt J, Bleyer A. 2002. Late Effects of Childhood Cancer and Its Treatment. Pizzo PA, Poplack DG, Eds. *Principles and Practice of Pediatric Oncology.* 4th ed. Philadelphia: Lippincott Williams & Wilkins.

Erenberg A, Lemons J, Sia C, Trunkel D, Ziring P. 1999. Newborn and infant hearing loss: detection and intervention. American Academy of Pediatrics, task Force on newborn and Infant hearing, 1998-1999. *Pediatrics,* Feb, 103(2):527-30.

Ettinger A. 2002. *Long-Term Survivor Programs: A Paradigm for the Advanced Practice Nurse.* NCPB Commissioned Paper (*www.iom.edu/ncpb*).

Greenberg M. 2002. The Ontario Aftercare Program: Dawn of a New Era. *National Cancer Policy Board Meeting.* Washington, DC.

Harvey J, Hobbie WL, Shaw S, Bottomley S. 1999. Providing quality care in childhood cancer survivorship: learning from the past, looking to the future. *J Pediatr Oncol Nurs* 16(3):117-25.

Hobbie WL, Hollen PJ. 1993. Pediatric nurse practitioners specializing with survivors of childhood cancer. *J Pediatr Health Care* 7(1):24-30.

Hollen PJ, Hobbie WL. 1995. Establishing comprehensive specialty follow-up clinics for long-term survivors of cancer. Providing systematic physiological and psychosocial support. *Support Care Cancer* 3(1):40-4.

Kadan-Lottick NS, Robison LL, Gurney JG, Neglia JP, Yasui Y, Hayashi R, Hudson M, Greenberg M, Mertens AC. 2002. Childhood cancer survivors' knowledge about their past diagnosis and treatment: Childhood Cancer Survivor Study. *JAMA* 287(14):1832-9.

Keene N. 2002. Solicitation of concerns of cancer survivors and their family through survivorship listserv and provided to the National Cancer Policy Board.

Keene N, Hobbie W, Ruccione K. 2000. *Childhood Cancer Survivors: A Practical Guide to Your Future.* Sebastopol, CA: O'Reilly and Associates, Inc.

MacLean WE Jr, Foley GV, Ruccione K, Sklar C. 1996. Transitions in the care of adolescent and young adult survivors of childhood cancer. *Cancer* 78(6):1340-4.

Masera G, Chesler M, Jankovic M, Eden T, Nesbit ME, Van Dongen-Melman J, Epelman C, Ben Arush MW, Schuler D, Mulhern R. 1996. SIOP Working Committee on Psychosocial issues in pediatric oncology: guidelines for care of long-term survivors. *Med Pediatr Oncol* 27(1):1-2.

Mullen CA, Petropoulos D, Roberts WM, Rytting M, Zipf T, Chan KW, Culbert SJ, Danielson M, Jeha SS, Kuttesch JF, Rolston KV. 1999. Outpatient treatment of fever and neutropenia for low risk pediatric cancer patients. *Cancer* 86(1):126-34.

Murphy S. 2002. Clinical Trials: Issues Impacting Design and Conduct of Clinical Trials, NCPB Commissioned Paper. (*www.iom.edu/ncpb*).

National Ambulatory Medical Care Survey and National Hospital Ambulatory Medical Care Survey, 1995-1999; Healthcare Cost and Utilization Project, 1997; special tabulations NCPB staff, 2003.

Newacheck PW, Strickland B, Shonkoff JP, Perrin JM, McPherson M, McManus M, Lauver C, Fox H, Arango P. 1998. An epidemiologic profile of children with special health care needs. *Pediatrics* 102(1 Pt 1):117-23.

Oeffinger KC. 2002. Longitudinal Cancer-related Health Care for Adult Survivors of Childhood Cancer (IOM commissioned background paper) (*www.iom.edu/ncpb*).

Oeffinger KC, Eshelman DA, Tomlinson GE, Buchanan GR. 1998. Programs for adult survivors of childhood cancer. *J Clin Oncol* 16(8):2864-7.

Oeffinger KC, Mertens AC, Hudson MM, Gurney JG, Casillas J, Chen H, Yeazel M, Whitton J, Yasui Y, Robison LL. 2003. Health care of young adult survivors of childhood cancer: A report from the Childhood Cancer Survivor Study. *Annals of Family Medicine.*

Perrin EC, Starr MC. 1993. Pediatric chronic illness. *J Learn Disabil* 26(7):426-7.

Perrin JM. 2002. Health services research for children with disabilities. *Milbank Q* 80(2):303-24.

Pizzo PA. 1990. Cancer and the pediatrician: an evolving partnership. *Pediatr Rev* 12(1):5-6.

Ross JA, Severson RK, Robison LL, Pollock BH, Neglia JP, Woods WG, Hammond GD. 1993. Pediatric cancer in the United States. A preliminary report of a collaborative study of the Childrens Cancer Group and the Pediatric Oncology Group. *Cancer* 71(10 Suppl):3415-21.

Ross JA, Severson RK, Pollock BH, Robison LL. 1996. Childhood cancer in the United States. A geographical analysis of cases from the Pediatric Cooperative Clinical Trials groups. *Cancer* 77(1):201-7.

Schwartz C, Hobbie W, Constine L, Ruccione K. 1994. *Survivors of Childhood Cancer: Assessment and Management.* St. Louis, MO: Mosby.

Shochat SJ, Fremgen AM, Murphy SB, Hutchison C, Donaldson SS, Haase GM, Provisor AJ, Clive-Bumpus RE, Winchester DP. 2001. Childhood cancer: patterns of protocol participation in a national survey. *CA Cancer J Clin* 51(2):119-30.

Simone JV, Lyons J. 1998. The evolution of cancer care for children and adults. *J Clin Oncol* 16(9):2904-5.

Trabert, E. 2001. Long-term Follow-up Programs for Survivors of Childhood Cancer. National Cancer Policy Board Background Paper (*www.iom.edu/ncpb*).

Wallace WH, Blacklay A, Eiser C, Davies H, Hawkins M, Levitt GA, Jenney ME. 2001. Developing strategies for long term follow up of survivors of childhood cancer. *BMJ* 323(7307):271-4.

Winn R.J. 2002. Care of the Cancer Survivor: Role and Availability of Specialized Clinic Services: National Cancer Policy Board Commissioned Paper (*www.iom.edu/ncpb*).

Wittes, R.E. 2003. Therapies for cancer in children—past success, future challenges. *N Engl J Med* Feb 20; 348(8):747-9.

Wolfe LC. 1993. A model system. Integration of services for cancer treatment. *Cancer* 72(11 Suppl):3525-30.

Wollnik L. 1976. Management of the child with cancer on an outpatient basis. *Nurs Clin North Am* 11(1):33-48.

Ziring PR, Brazdziunas D, Cooley WC, Kastner TA, Kummer ME, Gonzalez de Pijem L, Quint RD, Ruppert ES, Sandler AD, Anderson WC, Arango P, Burgan P, Garner C, McPherson M, Michaud L, Yeargin-Allsopp M, Johnson CP, Wheeler LS, Nackashi J, Perrin JM. 1999. American Academy of Pediatrics. Committee on Children with Disabilities. Care coordination: integrating health and related systems of care for children with special health care needs. *Pediatrics* 104(4 Pt 1):978-81.

6

Assuring Appropriate Educational Support Services

Going back to school or work following cancer treatment can signal a return to normalcy. Some survivors of childhood cancer are, however, left with persistent late effects of treatment that may interfere with their ability to receive an education or obtain gainful employment. Neurocognitive deficits, functional and sensory limitations, and symptoms such as fatigue are examples of late effects that can hamper educational and vocational success. Prolonged absence from school during illness may also slow educational progress and keep survivors from advancing to higher grade levels along with their peers.

This chapter first briefly reviews the prevalence of school-related disabilities among survivors of childhood cancer. Next, programs are described that are designed to assist cancer survivors and their families in reentry into school following treatment. The chapter concludes with a brief review of federal laws that protect the educational and employment rights of individuals with disabilities. This chapter draws heavily upon a review of educational issues for children with cancer published in 2002 (Leigh and Miles, 2002). In addition, two background papers commissioned by the Board were helpful in preparing this chapter, "Cognitive Late Effects of Childhood Cancer and Treatment: Issues for Survivors," by F. Daniel Armstrong, and "Policy Recommendations to Address the Employment and Insurance Concerns of Cancer Survivors," by Barbara Hoffman (*www. iom.edu/ncpb*). See Chapter 4 for a review of cognitive late effects, their implications for school achievement, and the limited research on interventions to ameliorate cognitive late effects.

DISABILITIES AMONG SCHOOL-AGE CANCER SURVIVORS

An estimated 5.5 percent of school-age children and adolescents (age 5 to 17) in the general population have chronic health conditions or impairments that contribute to an inability to attend school at all (0.6 percent), a need for special school or classes (3.7 percent), or a limitation in the amount of school attendance (1.2 percent) (Wenger,1995). There are few estimates of the proportion of survivors of childhood cancer with limitations that may affect school performance. Educational outcomes among survivors of acute lymphoblastic leukemia (ALL) and central nervous system (CNS) tumors have been assessed because they are generally exposed to treatments that can affect neurocognitive function (see Chapter 4). These cancers make up about 50 to 60 percent of newly diagnosed cases of childhood cancer and so, represent a significant share of the survivorship population. The largest study of educational outcomes to date suggests that ALL survivors have lower grades, enroll in special education or learning disability programs at three to four times the rate of their siblings, and when enrolled in such programs, spend a longer time in them as compared with their siblings. ALL survivors are also at higher risk of missing school for long periods and of repeating a year of school. On the other hand, most ALL survivors had rates of high school graduation, college entry, and college graduation that were similar to those of their brothers and sisters. Only survivors treated with 24 Gy of cranial radiation and those diagnosed at a preschool age were at higher risk for poor educational performance (Haupt et al., 1994) (see Chapter 4 and Table 4.3 for details of this study). The cohort of survivors treated in the 1970s and 1980s were at especially high risk for school-related problems because many of them were treated with 24 Gy of radiation. Few children with ALL now receive doses of cranial radiation this high, but the effects on school performance of treatment regimens common in the 1990s that relied on higher doses of chemotherapy have not yet been determined.

Among the general population, an estimated 11.2 percent of school-age children (age 6 to 17) are enrolled in federally sponsored special education programs (Department of Education, 2001).[1] Roughly 30 to 40 percent of

---

[1]The percentage of school-age children enrolled in federally sponsored special education programs (11.2 percent) is higher than the earlier mentioned estimate of children and adolescents with a chronic health condition or impairment and a disability related to schooling (5.5 percent). Many children enrolled in special education programs have learning disabilities that may not have been considered a chronic health condition or impairment in the survey from which the lower estimate was derived.

ALL survivors would be expected to be in special education programs if the three- to fourfold increase in use of special educational programs among survivors of ALL documented by Haupt and colleagues can be applied to survivors treated after the mid-1980s (Haupt et al., 1994). Other survivors of childhood cancer may not experience neurocognitive late effects, but need special accommodations because of physical limitations that impede participation in school-related activities. Irrespective of education placement upon reentering school following diagnosis and treatment, childhood cancer survivors and their families, teachers, and classmates can benefit from special transition services.

SCHOOL REENTRY INTERVENTIONS

Children are often absent from their regular school during periods of treatment and generally receive at least some educational services at home or in the hospital. School districts nationally vary tremendously in their guidelines for providing such services, the amount of weekly teaching provided (from a few hours per week to daily contacts), and in the preparation and familiarity of teachers in these settings to meet complex educational needs during limited teaching contacts. A child's educational experience may lack continuity if he or she goes back and forth between hospitalizations and home and/or school over the course of treatment.

A return to their familiar school and classmates following treatment can be a long- awaited event, but can also raise fears about peer teasing or the ability to resume a pre-cancer level of activity and function. A school with 500 to 1,000 students may have a student with cancer enrolled every few years, but given the rarity of new cases of childhood cancer, most teachers would not be expected to be familiar with the physical and psychosocial issues related to childhood cancer. Teachers may become more familiar with these issues as the number of childhood cancer survivors increases.

Organized educational programs for teachers and classmates have been successful in reducing problems associated with school reentry (Leigh and Miles, 2002). A well-defined and planned hospital/school program is necessary for hospitals, according to the International Society of Paediatric Oncology (SIOP) Working Committee on Psychosocial Issues in Pediatric Oncology (Masera et al., 1995). Programs vary in their approaches, but a general plan for school reentry has been described (Box 6.1).

Children may experience emotional, behavioral, or social problems at school reentry, may have physical needs (e.g., related to fatigue, mobility problems), and may have cognitive effects of treatment (Loman and Vincent, 2002). Children at highest academic risk include children with CNS-involved disease, a history of school problems, numerous or extended absences, and children who speak English as a second language (Loman and Vincent, 2002). Relatively little is known about the availability of school reentry programs, but a survey conducted from November 2001 through spring 2002 of 238 Children's Oncology Group (COG) institutions (55 percent response rate; 130 institutions) indicates that fewer than half of responding institutions (42 percent) had a formal program and roughly half (52 percent) had some services. Most programs had support from the hospital or department (54 percent) and from donations or grants (20 percent). Programs often provided (Loman and Vincent, 2002):

- home tutoring,
- communication between school, medical team and family,
- education for parents and children regarding going back to school,
- school staff consultation at the time of reentry,
- advocacy information for parents and individual education plan (IEP) help,
  - neuropsychological evaluations,[2]
  - individual or family therapy, and
  - class presentations.

Another study of support services available to cancer survivors within National Cancer Institute (NCI)-designated comprehensive cancer centers found only 7 of 37 (19 percent) centers with school re-entry programs (Tesauro et al., 2002).

Most of the school-based educational programs that are responsive to the needs of survivors of childhood cancer are in place following the enactment of federal laws to protect the educational and employment rights of individuals with disabilities.

FEDERAL LAWS AND PROGRAMS[3]

Three federal laws protect the educational and employment rights of individuals with disabilities:

- the Individuals with Disabilities Education Act (IDEA) of 1975 and IDEA amendments of 1997 support states to ensure the provision of free appropriate public education of children with disabilities (age 3 to 21);

---

[2]Neuropsychological evaluations were provided by nearly two-thirds of institutions.

[3]Much of this section is excerpted directly from the chapter in *Principle and Practices of Pediatric Oncology*, "Educational Issues for Children with Cancer" (Chapter 50) by Leigh and Miles (2000).

Box 6.1
Phases of School Reentry for Children with Cancer

Phase 1: Initial hospitalization and plans for reentry

As a first step, a hospital-based school liaison should be identified soon after diagnosis to work with parents as an advocate for the child and to serve as a bridge between the hospital and school personnel. The importance of a child's returning to school and to other normal activities should be discussed early as part of the treatment plan by physicians. Schools are responsible for providing a teacher for instruction if a child is home-bound or in the hospital and close to school. The school district in which the hospital is located may be responsible for providing education for children being cared for far from home. Some school systems lend laptop computers to students who are hospitalized so that they can use e-mail to send assignments and maintain communication with classmates. Other technologies that may be available include video teleconferencing with a child's classroom and the use of computer programs and the Internet. With the parent's permission, the school liaison can work with the teacher, counselor, or both to provide appropriate information to an affected child's classmates about the diagnosis and the anticipated length of absence from school. Factors that can affect educational outcomes should be documented including information on any pre-existing learning disabilities or chronic illness, and the specific nature of the cancer and its treatment. Neurocognitive testing begins before treatment and plans should be made for repeated assessment to detect emerging treatment-related disabilities that may not be seen for several years after treatment.

Phase 2: Contact and education of school personnel

All children should be given the opportunity to express their individual concerns and information should be provided about services available to assist them upon

• the Rehabilitation Act (section 504) provides a broader set of protections for individuals of all ages with disabilities to ensure that discrimination does not occur within any program in receipt of federal funds.

• the Americans with Disabilities Act (ADA) prohibits discrimination of persons with disabilities of all ages in both public and privately supported agencies and business and requires that persons with disabilities receive reasonable accommodation.

These laws apply to every level of education, from preschool to college and vocational education. Although these laws are federal, local and state governments interpret and implement them differently (Root et al., 1993). Any services needed by children in school, such as special education or classroom accommodations, have to be identified in a formal written plan according to specifications in the IDEA or in section 504 of the Rehabilitation Act. The written, signed plan protects affected children's rights and their return to school. A presentation about illness and treatment to classmates or teachers can provide children and classmates with examples of what can be said or how situations can be handled. Parents need reassurance to assuage fears, for example, that their child will be exposed to infections or that they will not be able to cope. Parental reactions, such as separation anxiety, may need to be assessed. An interview with teachers can help them appreciate realistic academic expectations of the returning student and prepare them for the psychosocial issues that may emerge following school reentry. Peer education may ease misconceptions regarding cancer, aid classmates in their desire to be helpful, and forestall teasing or other inappropriate behaviors.

Phase 3: Follow-up contact

Frequent communication between school personnel and the school liaison should continue following school reentry to assess how children are adjusting to the school environment and to ensure the receipt of appropriate educational and supportive services. A schedule of follow-up testing for high-risk children is recommended because neurocognitive deficits may not appear until 2 to 4 years following treatment. In the long term, transitional services to support college entry or vocational training may be appropriate if accommodations are needed because of a learning or other disability. For terminally ill children, continued school participation may also be important. School participation can change from school attendance to home-bound services or any combination of the two to accommodate terminally ill children's physical problems or minimize their discomfort. At some time, academics will no longer be appropriate, and teachers may want to engage children in other activities. Mental health consultation may be needed to support not only the child and their caregivers, but also teachers and classmates.

SOURCE: Adapted from Leigh and Miles, 2002.

provides documentation needed by parents if the services are not provided appropriately.

Individuals with Disabilities Education Act

The Individuals with Disabilities Education Act (IDEA) (20 U.S.C. 1400 et seq.) establishes a federal grant program to assist states in providing children with disabilities with a "free, appropriate public education which includes special education and related services, to meet the unique needs of all disabled individuals between the age of three and 21" (34 Code of Federal Regulation [CFR], Sec. 300.1[a]). Special education is defined as "specially designed instruction, at no cost to the parents, to meet the needs of a child with a disability" (34 CFR, Sec. 300.17). Special education includes services ranging from simple classroom accommodations in a regular classroom to all-day placement in a resource room environment to instruction in the home, hospital, or other institution. Related services refers to transportation, corrective, and other supportive services that are required for children with a disability to benefit from special education. These include audiology and speech pathology, psychological services, physical and occupational therapy, recreation, counseling services, school health services, social work services in schools, and parent counseling and training (34 CFR, Sec. 300.16). Available classroom accommodations may include use of a scribe or tape recorder to take notes, shortened class or homework assignments, provision of information instead of copying from a board or book, preferential seating, more time for tests or written work, oral testing, and permission to leave class early to avoid accidental injury caused by travel through crowded hallways. Although schools are not required to provide all medical services, they must provide certain medical services that are necessary to implement the IEP. For example, a child who uses a catheter is entitled to the services of a school nurse or other trained personnel to help keep the catheter clean during the school day.

Education must be provided in the least restrictive setting and where possible, school districts are required to provide children with disabilities an education in the regular classroom setting. To receive special education services under provisions of the IDEA, children must meet criteria for classification under at least one of several categories: mental retardation, hearing impairment, vision impairment, speech or language impairment, serious emotional disturbance, autism, deaf-blindness, traumatic brain injury, specific learning disability, orthopedic impairment, other health impairment, or multiple disabilities. Most children with cancer are eligible for services under the category "other health impairment," defined as "a child who has limited strength, vitality, or alertness due to chronic or acute health problems, such as heart condition, tuberculosis, rheumatic fever, nephritis, asthma, sickle cell anemia, hemophilia, epilepsy, lead poisoning, leukemia, or diabetes which adversely affects educational performance" (34 CFR, Sec. 300.7). A physician often completes a form to verify the diagnosis, treatment, and related impairments to facilitate the eligibility determination process. Eligibility for services are, in part, determined by evaluations of aptitude and achievement. Eligibility for IDEA services under the category specific learning disability requires a discrepancy of one standard deviation (15 points) between measured intelligence quotient and measured academic achievement. For children treated for cancer, this discrepancy may not show up for years and for that reason, many children with cancer receive services under the IDEA category "other health impairment" or under section 504 of the Rehabilitation Act (see discussion below). These categories for eligibility do not require the use of a discrepancy score.

Under IDEA, reassessments are made every three years. However, evidence suggests that neurocognitive testing to identify deficits following treatment of ALL or CNS tumors should be conducted more frequently with the timing and intensity of testing determined by the child's age at the time of treatment, interval since treatment, and anticipated potential areas of difficulty based on typical developmental trajectories (Armstrong, 2002). Thus, for some children, evaluations every 12 to 18 months may be necessary during periods of rapid development, and for others, evaluations every 2 to 3 years may be adequate during periods of less rapid development. Although a psychologist with expertise in the appropriate psychometric tools may be needed to administer and interpret these tests, third party payers usually do not cover the cost of testing outside of the school system.

If a child is determined to be eligible for services, an individual education plan (IEP) is designed by a multidisciplinary group of school staff, parents, and sometimes, the child. After the IEP is signed by all participants at the meeting, it becomes a legal document that, by law, the state must carry out as written. The goals and objectives of the IEP are reviewed annually, and the IEP is rewritten if necessary. Every 3 years, the child is reassessed. Beginning at age 14, each student's IEP must include specific transition-related content and beginning no later than age 16, a statement of needed transition services. Transition services are defined as "a coordinated set of activities for a student, designed within an outcome-oriented process, that promotes movement from school to post-school activities, including post-secondary education, vocational training, integrated employment (including supported employment), continuing and adult education, adult services, independent living, or community participation. The coordinated set of activities must be based on the individual student's needs, taking into account the student's preferences and interests; and must include needed activities in the areas of instruction, community experiences, the development of employment and other post-school adult living objectives and, if appropriate, acquisition of daily living skills and functional vocational evaluation" (34 CFR, Sec. 300.29).

The IDEA also mandates early intervention services for infants and toddlers who are either disabled or at risk of developmental delays. These services are provided either by school systems or by the state health department.

Parents have specific rights under IDEA, including a request for review and modification of the IEP. This can also be requested by the school system. The school system is required to attempt full implementation of the IEP, but there are no specified consequences for non-implementation. Parents have a right to seek a legal remedy to ensure compliance with the IEP. Anecdotal reports suggest that satisfaction with the IEP process and related services is highly variable, and depends on the level of cooperation provided by the school, the school system's awareness of cognitive impairment in

children with cancer, and resources available to provide the necessary interventions (Hoffman, 2002). Accessing special education services under IDEA
can be a complex undertaking and some parents benefit from training to
become an educational advocate for their child. Parental advocacy skills
are critical, especially when families live far from their child's treating
facility or when parents need to overcome language and cultural-related
difficulties in negotiating through complex school programs. The Department of Education supports parent centers in each state that provide training and information to help parents participate more effectively with
professionals in meeting the education needs of children and youth with
disabilities (*www.taalliance.org/PTIs.htm*, accessed March 15, 2003). Cancer centers may also provide parent training on the basics of special education services, how IEPs should be tailored to the specific needs of their
child, how to appeal limitations on educational services offered to a child,
and how to get help from organizations such as Candlelighters and local
legal aid societies when services are designated but not provided, or provided in an ineffective manner. In some areas, ombudsman programs are
available to provide an advocate to attend the IEP session with a parent to
help negotiate for needed services.

The Rehabilitation Act of 1973

Section 504 of the Rehabilitation Act of 1973 (re-authorized in 1998)
"clarifies that no individual with a disability in the United States, shall,
solely by reason of his or her disability, be excluded from the participation
in, be denied the benefits of, or be subjected to discrimination under any
program or activity receiving Federal financial assistance or any program or
activity conducted by any Executive agency" (34 CFR, Sec. 104.4). Program or activity is defined as including "all operations of a local education
agency, system of vocational education, or other school system." This law
applies also to colleges, universities, and private schools that receive federal
funds. Under the provisions of this law, the definition of disability is
broader: "a physical or mental impairment which substantially limits one
or more of such person's major life activities, such as learning; a record of
such an impairment; or being regarded as having such an impairment."
The pertinent disability is not required to affect school performance adversely, and affected children do not have to come under the umbrella of
special education to receive services. All persons at any age with diagnosed
cancer are eligible to receive services under section 504. For affected children to receive services, a meeting similar to that for an IEP is conducted,
and the needed services are written in the form of what is called a 504 plan.
Unlike the IEP process however, a 504 plan is not monitored for compliance and does not have to be reviewed annually.

In addition to stipulating conditions in academic settings, the Rehabilitation Act prohibits discrimination in employment practices; program accessibility; health, welfare, and other social services; nonacademic and extracurricular activities, including clubs; counseling services; transportation; and health services.

Americans with Disabilities Act

The ADA of 1990 provides a wider range of protection for all persons with disabilities. It prohibits discrimination against persons with disabilities and applies to all state and local agencies (not just those receiving federal funds), including private businesses. The ADA mandates that no individual with a disability shall be excluded from participation in public services or programs, such as higher education (42 U.S.C. 12132). The ADA not only prohibits discrimination against persons with disabilities, but requires that persons with disabilities receive "reasonable accommodation." Its provisions apply to education, including non-sectarian private schools. It provides a second layer of protection, in addition to section 504, to ensure that public schools provide reasonable accommodations for students with disabilities. For example, a university may be required to provide a sign-language interpreter to a cancer survivor who has a hearing loss as a result of treatment. Additionally, the institution may not discriminate on the basis of the student's disability. For example, a survivor who has respiratory fibrosis may not be required to complete the same physical educational standards required of other students.

How effective are special education programs in addressing the needs of childhood cancer survivors? Unfortunately, there are no data to document specific outcomes (e.g., maintenance of developmental trajectories or improvement in functioning) for childhood cancer survivors who are provided with standardized access to special education services. Intervention studies are underway to assess programs designed to improve neurocognitive outcomes among survivors of childhood cancer (Armstrong, 2002). These interventions include improving the academic and social reintegration of children into the school setting; training parents to be more effective advocates for their child's educational needs; and evaluating specific behavioral, medical, and compensatory interventions.

SUMMARY AND CONCLUSIONS

School-related disabilities among survivors of childhood cancer may include learning disabilities and functional limitations. There are no good estimates of how many childhood cancer survivors need accommodations at school, but among certain groups of survivors, the need appears to be very high. There is, for example, a three- to fourfold increase in the use of special education services among survivors of ALL, which likely translates into a third to a half of such survivors needing special education programs. Survivors at higher risk for neurocognitive late effects require monitoring for long-term neurocognitive deficits that may arise in the years following treatment. More needs to be learned of the educational needs of other groups of childhood cancer survivors and of the effectiveness of interventions designed to ameliorate the late effects of cancer and its treatment.

Many cancer centers have school programs to ease the return of childhood cancer survivors to school following their treatment. Ideally, planning for school reentry begins at diagnosis and involves a school liaison to ensure that educational environments are supportive and can accommodate any late effects. The school liaison's role may include following the educational progress of survivors through transitions to college, employment, or vocational programs. Support to teachers and classmates may also be provided following the death of a child from cancer.

Three federal laws protect the educational and employment rights of individuals with disabilities: IDEA, the Rehabilitation Act of 1973, and the ADA. IDEA supports states to ensure the provision of free appropriate public education of children with disabilities. The Rehabilitation Act provides a broader set of protections for individuals of all ages with disabilities, to ensure that discrimination does not occur within any program in receipt of federal funds. The ADA prohibits discrimination of persons of disabilities in both public and privately supported agencies and business and requires that persons with disabilities receive reasonable accommodation. Of most direct relevance to children with cancer and their families is the IDEA and the protections afforded by the Rehabilitation Act of 1973. While legal protections appear to be comprehensive, required procedures are implemented and legal interpretations are made locally. Consequently, among parents, satisfaction with accommodations at schools varies, depending on the school's level of cooperation, awareness of cognitive impairment in children with cancer, and resources available to provide the necessary interventions.

REFERENCES

Armstrong D. F. 2002. Cognitive Late Effects of Childhood Cancer and Treatment: Issues for Survivors (IOM commissioned background paper) (*www.iom.edu/ncpb*).

Haupt R, Fears TR, Robison LL, Mills JL, Nicholson HS, Zeltzer LK, Meadows AT, Byrne J. 1994. Educational attainment in long-term survivors of childhood acute lymphoblastic leukemia. *JAMA* 272(18):1427-32.

Hoffman B. 2002. Policy Recommendations to Address the Employment and Insurance Concerns of Cancer Survivors (IOM commissioned background paper) (*www.iom.edu/ncpb*).

Leigh LD, Miles MA. 2002. Educational Issues for Children with Cancer. Pizzo PA, Poplack DG. *Principles and Practice of Pediatric Oncology.* 4th ed. Philadelphia: Lippicott Williams and Wilkins. Pp. 1463-76.

Loman P, Vincent N. 2002. School Reintegration: Current Trends and Future Directions. Presentation at a meeting of the Children's Oncology Group, St. Louis, MO (October 2002).

Masera G, Jankovic M, Deasy-Spinetta P, Adamoli L, Ben Arush MW, Challinor J, Chesler M, Colegrove R, Van Dongen-Melman J, McDowell H, et al. 1995. SIOP Working Committee on Psychosocial Issues in Pediatric Oncology: guidelines for school/education. *Med Pediatr Oncol* 25(6):429-30.

Root H, Deasy-Spinetta P, Fiduccia D, et al. 1993. Protection of Children's Educational Rights. Deasy-Spinetta P, Irvin E, eds. *Educating the Child With Cancer.* Bethesda, MD: The Candlelighter's Childhood Cancer Foundation.

Tesauro GM, Rowland JH, Lustig C. 2002. Survivorship resources for post-treatment cancer survivors. *Cancer Pract* 10(6):277-83.

U.S. Department of Education. 2001. *Twenty-Third Annual Report to Congress on the Implementation of the Individuals with Disabilities Act.* Washington, DC: U.S. Department of Education.

Wenger BL, Kaye HS, La Plante MP. Disabilities Among Children. 1995. *Disability Statistics Abstract No. 15.* Washington, DC: U.S. Department of Education, National Institute on Disability and Rehabilitation Research.

7

Employment, Insurance, and Economic Issues

A history of cancer can have a significant impact on employment opportunities and may also affect being able to obtain and retain health and life insurance (Ferrell and Hassey Dow, 1997; Monaco et al., 1997; President's Cancer Panel, 2001; Weiner et al., 2002). This chapter outlines the employment and insurance concerns of particular relevance to survivors of childhood cancer.[1] The current legal remedies to these socioeconomic problems are described, as are potential educational, legislative, and advocacy responses. Selected federal and state programs are described that are of relevance to childhood cancer survivors, including Medicaid and Medicare, Supplemental Security Income (SSI), Social Security Disability Insurance (SSDI), and the Title V Children with Special Health Care Needs (CSHCN) program.

EMPLOYMENT

The Impact of Cancer on Survivors' Employment Opportunities

Most cancer survivors who worked before their diagnosis return to work following their treatment (Crothers, 1986). Retaining one's employ-

---

[1]Much of this chapter is based on a background paper prepared by Barbara Hoffman and material from *A Cancer Survivor's Almanac: Charting Your Journey*. There are no commercial genetic screening tests available to predict pediatric cancer or cancer recurrence among survivors of pediatric cancer and so the potential for discrimination on the basis of genetic testing is not discussed.

ment status has obvious financial benefits and is often also necessary for health insurance coverage, self-esteem, and social support. Survivors of childhood cancer may have late effects that limit their initial entry into the workforce or restrict their employment options. In a recent study of over 10,000 members of the Childhood Cancer Survivor Study cohort, virtually all (95 percent) of the survivors had worked, but the likelihood of employment was lower as compared to their siblings (Pang et al., 2002). Similar findings emerged from an earlier survey of 219 childhood survivors who were treated between 1945 and 1975 and were at least 30 years old at the time of the survey. Childhood survivors, with the exception of survivors of CNS tumors, reported very similar employment histories as a matched control group. Members of the control group, however, reported somewhat higher annual incomes than did the survivors (Hays et al., 1992).

When employed, cancer survivors have often reported problems in the workplace, including dismissal, failure to hire, demotion, denial of promotion, undesirable transfer, denial of benefits, and hostility (Hoffman, 1996). Studies conducted prior to the passage of comprehensive employment discrimination laws suggest that survivors of childhood cancer encountered substantial employment obstacles:

• 43 of 403 (11 percent) Hodgkin's disease survivors treated at Stanford University experienced difficulties at work that they attributed to their cancer history (Fobair et al., 1986),
• approximately 11 percent of adult survivors of childhood cancer reported some form of employment-related discrimination according to a study of 227 former pediatric cancer patients (Green et al., 1991),
• 15 of 60 (25 percent) survivors of childhood cancer in another study reported job discrimination (10 persons were refused a job at least once, 3 were denied benefits, 3 experienced illness-related conflict with a supervisor, 4 reported job task problems, and 11 were rejected by the military) (Koocher and O'Malley, 1982),
• 8 of the 40 (20 percent) survivors of childhood/adolescent Hodgkin's disease reported job problems (Wasserman et al., 1987), and
• younger cancer survivors who were either employed or active in the labor market were more concerned than older survivors about revealing their cancer history in searching for another job (Koocher and O'Malley, 1982).

Most employers treat cancer survivors fairly and legally. Some employers, however, erect unnecessary and sometimes illegal barriers to survivors' job opportunities (Hoffman, 1996; Hoffman, 1999; Hoffman, 2002a). Most personnel decisions are driven by economic factors, not by charitable or personal consideration. Employers may be motivated to fire an employee with cancer (or a history of cancer) because of concerns about increased costs due to insurance expenses and lost productivity or because of concerns about the psychological impact of a survivors' cancer history on other employees. Some employers may fail to revise their personnel policies to comply with new laws, and even among those with updated policies, employers may not train their personnel managers properly to comply with these laws. The interpretation of laws designed to prohibit discriminatory practices is sometimes unclear and is being resolved in the courts. Some employers and co-workers treat cancer survivors differently from other workers, in part, because they have misconceptions about survivors' abilities to work during and after cancer treatment (Working Woman/ Amgen, 1996; Yankelovich, 1992).

Cancer Survivors' Current Employment Rights

Although cancer survivors do not have an unqualified right to obtain and retain employment, they do have the right to some freedom from discrimination and to be treated according to their individual abilities. Three federal laws—the Americans with Disabilities Act, the Family and Medical Leave Act, and the Employee Retirement and Income Security Act—provide cancer survivors with some protection against employment discrimination.

Americans with Disabilities Act

The Americans with Disabilities Act (ADA) of 1990 (42 U.S.C. 12101 et seq.) prohibits some types of job discrimination by employers, employment agencies, and labor unions against people who have or have had cancer. All private employers with 15 or more employees, state and local governments, the legislative branch of the federal government, employment agencies, and labor unions are covered by the ADA.

A "qualified individual with a disability" is protected by the ADA if he or she can perform the "essential functions" of the job. The ADA prohibits employment discrimination against individuals with a "disability," a "record" of a "disability," or who are "regarded" as having a "disability." A "disability" is a major health "impairment" that substantially limits the ability to do everyday activities, such as drive a car or go to work.

Cancer is an "impairment" as defined by the law. In most circumstances, cancer survivors, regardless of whether they are in treatment, in remission, or cured, are protected as persons with a disability because their cancer substantially limited a major life activity. Indeed, many federal courts and the Equal Employment Opportunities Commission (EEOC) consider cancer in most circumstances to be a disability under the ADA

(Hoffman, 2000). Whether a cancer survivor is covered by the ADA is determined, however, on a case-by-case basis. Because the United States Supreme Court has not, to date, squarely addressed whether *all* cancer survivors are protected by the ADA, cancer survivors' rights under the law vary depending on the facts of the individual case and the court in which the case is heard. Some courts have concluded that cancer survivors are "persons with a disability" as defined by the statute. Other courts, however, have placed cancer survivors in a "Catch-22" by concluding that a cancer survivor who is sufficiently healthy to work is not a person with a disability as defined by the ADA. In one case a woman with breast cancer was acknowledged to have experienced nausea, fatigue, swelling, inflammation, and pain resulting from her treatment, but the United States Court of Appeals for the Fifth Circuit found that she could nonetheless perform her essential job duties with accommodations (*Ellison v. Software Spectrum Inc.*). Although the Court of Appeals found that the woman's cancer affected her ability to work, it concluded that these limitations were not sufficient to render her a "person with a disability" as defined by the ADA. Other courts have followed the reasoning of the Fifth Circuit and rejected lawsuits by cancer survivors. In another case, a long-term survivor of non-Hodgkin's lymphoma, fired because his employer feared that future health insurance claims would cause his insurance costs to rise, was determined not to be covered under the ADA after his dismissal (*Hirsch v. National Mall and Serv., Inc.*). The court concluded "that the ADA was not truly meant to apply to this situation" because the claimant was discriminated against due to the costs of his cancer treatment, and not because of the cancer itself" (989 F. Supp. 977, 980).

The ADA prohibits discrimination in most job-related activities such as hiring, firing, and benefits. In most cases, a prospective employer may not ask applicants if they have ever had cancer. An employer has the right to know only if an applicant is able to perform the essential functions of the job. A job offer may be contingent upon passing a relevant medical exam, provided that all prospective employees are subject to the same exam. An employer may ask detailed questions about health only after making a job offer.

Cancer survivors who need extra time or help to work are entitled to a "reasonable accommodation." Common accommodations for survivors include changes in work hours or duties to accommodate medical appointments and treatment side effects. An employer does not have to make changes that would impose an "undue hardship" on the business or other workers. "Undue hardship" refers to any accommodation that would be unduly costly, extensive, substantial or disruptive, or that would fundamentally alter the nature or operation of the business. For example, an employer may replace a survivor who has to miss six months of work that cannot be performed by a temporary employee.

The ADA does not prohibit an employer from ever firing or refusing to hire a cancer survivor. Because the law requires employers to treat all employees similarly, regardless of disability, an employer may fire a cancer survivor who would have been terminated even if he or she was not a survivor.

Most employment discrimination laws protect only the employee. The ADA offers protection more responsive to survivors' needs because it prohibits discrimination against family members, too. Employers may not discriminate against workers because of their relationship or association with a "disabled" person. Employers may not assume that an employee's job performance would be affected by the need to care for a family member who has cancer.

Family and Medical Leave Act

The Family and Medical Leave Act (FMLA) (29 U.S.C. 2601 et seq.) requires employers with at least 50 workers to provide certain benefits for serious medical illness, including cancer, for employees or dependents. The statute provides a number of benefits to cancer survivors:

- provides 12 weeks of unpaid leave during any 12 month period,
- requires employers to continue to provide benefits, including health insurance coverage, during the leave period,
- requires employers to restore employees to the same or equivalent position at the end of the leave period,
- allows leave to care for a spouse, child, or parent who has a "serious health condition" such as cancer,
- allows leave because a serious health condition renders the employee "unable to perform the functions of the position,"
- allows intermittent or reduced work schedule when "medically necessary" (under some circumstances, an employer may transfer the employee to a position with equivalent pay and benefits to accommodate the new work schedule), and
- allows employees to "stack" or add leave under the FMLA to leave allowable under state medical leave law.

The FMLA reasonably balances the needs of the employer and employee. It

- requires employees to make reasonable efforts to schedule foreseeable medical care so as to not disrupt unduly the workplace,

- requires employees to give employers 30 days notice of foreseeable medical leave, or as much notice as is practicable,
- allows employers to require employees to provide certification of medical needs and allows employers to seek a second opinion, at the employer's expense, to corroborate medical need, and
- permits employers to provide leave provisions more generous than those required by the FMLA.

In addition to the ADA and FMLA, another federal law, the Employee Retirement and Income Security Act (ERISA) and an Executive Order provide some legal protection for cancer survivors who encounter problems at work.

The Employee Retirement and Income Security Act (ERISA)

The Employee Retirement and Income Security Act (29 U.S.C. 1001 et seq.) prohibits an employer from discriminating against an employee to prevent him or her from collecting benefits under an employee benefit plan. Employee benefit plans are defined broadly, and include any plan providing "medical, surgical, or hospital care benefits, or benefits in the event of sickness, accident, disability, death, or unemployment." Employers who offer group benefit packages to their employees are subject to ERISA. ERISA does not, however, apply to the large number of employers who self fund their insurance plans.

Some employers fear that the participation of a cancer survivor in a group medical plan will drain benefit funds or increase the employer's insurance premiums. An employer may violate ERISA if, upon learning of a worker's cancer history, it dismisses that worker to exclude him or her from a group health plan. An employer also may violate ERISA by encouraging a person with a cancer history to retire as a "disabled" employee. Most benefit plans define disability narrowly to include only the most debilitating conditions. Individuals with a cancer history often do not fit under such a definition and should not be compelled to so label themselves.

ERISA covers both participants (employees) and beneficiaries (spouses and children). Thus, if the employee is fired because his or her child has cancer, the employee may be entitled to file a claim. ERISA, however, is inapplicable to many victims of employment discrimination, including individuals who are denied a new job because of their medical status, employees who are subjected to differential treatment that does not affect their benefits, and employees whose compensation does not include benefits.

Executive Order

Unlike most private and state employees, federal employees are protected from genetic-based discrimination. An Executive Order issued by President Clinton in 2000 prohibits federal departments and agencies form making employment decisions about civilian federal employees based on protected genetic information (*http://www.opm.gov/pressrel/2000/genetic_eo.htm*, accessed March 15, 2003). The Order also prohibits federal employers from requiring genetic tests as a condition of being hired or receiving benefits.

State Employment Rights Laws

All states except Alabama and Mississippi have laws that prohibit discrimination against people with disabilities in public and private employment (Hoffman, 1996; Hoffman 2002a; Hoffman, personal communication to Maria hewitt, 2002). Alabama and Mississippi laws, which have not been amended since the 1970s, cover only state employees. Several states, such as New Jersey, cover all employers regardless of the number of employees. The laws in most states, however, cover only employers with a minimum number of employees. A few states, such as California and Vermont, expressly prohibit discrimination against cancer survivors. Many state laws protect individuals with real or perceived disabilities, and therefore, cover most cases of cancer-based discrimination. The rights of cancer survivors who do not have a physical or mental impairment (and would be considered non-"handicapped" in some states) are unclear in those states where courts have not addressed the issue.

Many states have leave laws similar to the federal FMLA in that they guarantee employees in the private sector unpaid leave for pregnancy, childbirth, and the adoption of a child. Some state laws provide employees with medical leave to address a serious illness, such as cancer. Several states provide coverage more extensive than the federal law.

State medical leave laws vary widely as to:

- how long an employee can take leave,
- which employees may take leave (most states require an employee to have worked for a minimum period of time),
- which employers must provide leave (a few states have leave laws that apply to employers of fewer than 50 employees),
- the definition of "family member" for whose illness an employee may take family medical leave,
- the type of illness that entitles an employee to medical leave,
- how much notice an employee must give prior to taking leave,

- whether an employee continues to receive benefits while on leave and who pays for them, and
- how the law is enforced (by state agency or through private lawsuit).

HEALTH INSURANCE

The Impact of Cancer on Health Insurance

Employment rights and health insurance rights are closely related because most adult Americans receive health insurance through an employer's group plan. Loss of health insurance may be secondary to loss of employment and employment discrimination. Many cancer survivors are unable to purchase affordable, effective coverage, especially those who are not covered by group policies. During the past decade, the way in which cancer survivors purchased and used health insurance, as well as the laws governing health insurance, have changed significantly (Hoffman, 1999).

Adult and childhood cancer survivors share many of the same problems in accessing and keeping health insurance. Several studies of survivors of adult cancer have disclosed barriers to insurance, including refusal of new applications, policy cancellations or reductions, higher premiums, waived or excluded pre-existing conditions, and extended waiting periods:

- Nearly one-half of Hodgkin's disease and leukemia survivors in one study reported insurance problems due to cancer. These problems include the denial of health insurance, increased insurance rates, problems changing from a group to an individual plan and lost health insurance (Kornblith et al., 1998).
- Approximately 25 percent of the 940 cancer patients surveyed by the Mayo Clinic Rehabilitation Program reported insurance "discrimination" (Crothers, 1986).
- Almost 30 percent of all employable cancer survivors in California reported encountering barriers to insurance (Burton and Jones, 1982).

Among survivors of childhood cancer, health insurance problems are compounded, because most survivors have only family-related insurance before the onset of cancer (Hays, 1993). Like survivors of adult cancer, the more years that have passed since treatment, the more likely it is that childhood cancer survivors can obtain health insurance on the same terms as nonsurvivors. Adolescents and young adults may be especially vulnerable to insurance problems. When adolescents turn between 19 and 23 years of age (depending on the state), they may have to leave their parents' or public insurance coverage and have few options for obtaining their own health insurance (White, 2002).

Several studies have documented insurance-related difficulties of childhood cancer survivors. In one study of 182 young adult survivors of childhood cancer in North Carolina, survivors were more likely than their siblings to be denied health insurance (25 vs 3 percent) and when insured were more likely to have pre-existing condition clauses in their health insurance policy (17 vs 12 percent) (Vann et al., 1995). In another study, adult long-term survivors of childhood cancer were covered by health insurance policies without cancer-related restrictions at similar rates to a control group (81 to 92 percent vs 82 to 95 percent) (Hays et al., 1992). Among survivors, 7 to 14 percent described difficulties experienced by their parents in obtaining affordable health insurance for the entire family during or after the survivor's illness (as compared with 5 to 10 percent of the controls) (Hays et al., 1992). In another study, 14 percent of male survivors of childhood cancer and 9 percent of female survivors of childhood cancer were rejected for health insurance (as compared with 1 percent and none among the controls) (Teta et al., 1986).

Cancer Survivors' Health Insurance Rights

Cancer survivors who have health insurance are entitled to all of the rights set forth in their policies. Insurers who fail to pay for treatment in accordance with the terms of the policies may be sued for violating the contract between the survivor and the insurer. Some survivors have successfully sued their insurers for breach of contract for failing to pay for chemotherapy, bone marrow transplants, and other treatment. Some survivors find that their policies have inadequate coverage for needed services. A health insurance policy may, for example, cover one prosthesis a year, but a growing adolescent may require more than one. Some survivors may have coverage for a needed service (e.g., neurocognitive testing), but the specialists needed to deliver it may not be available within a plan's network of providers (John Fontanesi, Professor, University of California, San Diego, personal communication to Maria Hewitt, November 12, 2002). State and federal laws offer cancer survivors very limited remedies to overcome barriers in securing adequate health insurance coverage.

Among those with insurance, there may be difficulties in getting reimbursement for interventions designed to prevent or ameliorate late effects of childhood cancer because of variations in the scope of benefits offered by plans. In a 1998 review of pediatric care coverage rules (i.e., medical necessity standards) specified in contracts of large commercial insurers, relatively few contracts (4 percent of those reviewed) were found to allow for services to prevent conditions, impairments, or disabilities (Fox and McManus, 2001).

Federal Health Insurance Laws

Four federal laws provide survivors some opportunities to keep health insurance that they obtain through work.

Americans with Disabilities Act   As noted above, the ADA (42 U.S.C. 12101 et seq.) prohibits employers from denying health insurance to cancer survivors if other employees with similar jobs receive insurance. The ADA does not require employers to provide health insurance, but when they choose to provide health insurance, they must do so fairly. An employer who does not provide a cancer survivor with the same health insurance provided to employees with similar jobs must prove that the failure to provide insurance is based on legitimate actuarial data or that the insurance plan would become bankrupt or suffer a drastic increase in premiums, co-payments, or deductibles. An employer, such as a small business, who can prove that it is unable to obtain an insurance policy to cover the survivor, may not have to provide the survivor with the same health benefits provided to other employees. Because the ADA protects employees from discrimination based on their "association" with a person with a disability, an employer may not refuse to provide a family health policy solely because one of the employee's dependents has cancer.

Health Insurance Portability and Accountability Act (HIPAA)   HIPPA helps cancer survivors retain their health insurance by:

- Alleviating "job-lock" by allowing individuals who have been insured for at least 12 months to change to a new job without losing coverage, even if they previously have been diagnosed with cancer. In addition, for previously uninsured individuals, group plans cannot impose pre-existing condition exclusions of more than 12 months for conditions for which medical advice, diagnosis, or treatment was received or recommended within the previous six months.
- Preventing group health plans from denying coverage based on health status factors such as current and past health, claims experience, medical history, and genetic information. Insurers, however, may uniformly exclude coverage for specific conditions and place lifetime caps on benefits.
- Increasing insurance portability for people changing from a group policy to an individual one.
- Requiring insurers of small groups to cover all interested small em-

ployers and to accept every eligible individual under the employer's plan who applies for coverage when first eligible.

• Requiring health plans to renew coverage for groups and individuals in most cases.

• Increasing the tax deduction for health insurance expenses available to self-employed individuals.

The Consolidated Omnibus Budget Reconciliation Act of 1986 (COBRA)
COBRA (PL 99-272) requires employers to offer group medical coverage to employees and their dependents who otherwise would have lost their group coverage due to individual circumstances. Public and private employers with more than 20 employees are required to make continued insurance coverage available to employees who quit, are terminated, or work reduced hours. Coverage must extend to surviving, divorced, or separated spouses, and to dependent children.

By allowing survivors to keep group insurance coverage for a limited time, COBRA provides valuable time to shop for long-term coverage. Although the survivor, and not the former employer, must pay for the continued coverage, the rate may not exceed by more than 2 percent the rate set for the survivor's former co-workers.

Eligibility for the employee, spouse, and dependent child varies under COBRA. The employee becomes eligible if he or she loses group health coverage because of a reduction in hours or because of termination due to reasons other than gross employee misconduct. The spouse of an employee becomes eligible for any of four reasons:

1) the death of a spouse,
2) termination of a spouse's employment (for reasons other than gross misconduct) or reduction in a spouse's hours of employment,
3) divorce or legal separation from a spouse, or
4) a spouse becomes eligible for Medicare.

The dependent child of an employee becomes eligible for any of five reasons:

1) the death of a parent,
2) the termination of a parent's employment or reduction in a parent's hours,
3) a parent's divorce or legal separation,
4) a parent becomes eligible for Medicare, or
5) a dependent ceases to be a "dependent child" under a specific group plan.

The continued coverage under COBRA must be identical to that offered to the families of the employee's former co-workers. If employment is terminated for any reason other than gross misconduct, the employee and his or her dependents can continue coverage for up to 18 months. A qualified beneficiary who is determined to be disabled for Social Security purposes at the time of the termination of employment or reduction in employment hours can continue COBRA coverage for a total of 29 months. Dependents can continue coverage for up to 36 months if their previous coverage will end because of any of the above reasons.

Continued coverage may be cut short if:

1) the employer no longer provides group health insurance to any of its employees,

2) the continuation coverage premium is not paid,

3) the survivor becomes covered under another group health plan, or

4) the survivor becomes eligible for Medicare.

ERISA As described earlier, ERISA prohibits an employer from discriminating against an employee to prevent him or her from collecting benefits under an employee group benefit plan. Employee benefit plans that are self-insured are regulated only by federal law, not state insurance law. Unlike commercial insurance plans that employers purchase to provide health insurance as a benefit for their employees, self-insured plans are funds set aside by employers to reimburse employees for their allowable medical expenses. Generally, large employer groups or unions find it to their benefit to self-insure, while smaller employer groups choose to finance employee health benefits through commercial insurers. The claims employees file to obtain their reimbursement through these plans are likely to be administered by commercial insurance companies, so most people covered through self-insured plans do not even realize their health insurance is somewhat different from insurance purchased through an insurance company.

State Insurance Laws

Every state regulates policies sold by insurance companies in the state. These laws vary significantly. Some states require insurance policies to cover off-label chemotherapy, minimum hospital stays for cancer surgery, and benefits for certain types of cancer treatment and screening. More than half the states operate high-risk insurance pools to help provide coverage to individuals who have been denied private health insurance in the individual market (Achman and Chollet, 2001). These high-risk pools are often used to comply with provisions in the Health Insurance Portability and Accountability Act that provide the right to convert a group health insurance policy to an individual policy. Some states enroll people who are eligible for Medicare in their high-risk pool so that they may obtain supplemental coverage. As of 2002, high-risk insurance pools covered about 153,000 people (DHHS press release, 2002).

According to a recent analysis, state high-risk pools have had a limited impact in making insurance available and affordable for otherwise uninsurable individuals. State risk pools often charge premiums that are high relative to incomes, and typically include sizable deductibles and copayments. Most risk pools limit lifetime benefits (e.g., $1 million in Missouri, Texas, Alabama) (Achman and Chollet, 2001)). Although high-risk pools are designed to meet the needs of people with serious or chronic illnesses, they often limit access by imposing waiting and "look-back" periods for preexisting conditions to reduce adverse selection. Enrollees who were diagnosed for treatment of a condition during a "look-back" period (typically 6 months) before enrolling in the pool are not covered for treatment of that condition during a specified waiting period after coverage (typically 6 months or a year) (Achman and Chollet, 2001). Some states have long waiting lists and others are closed to new applicants altogether (e.g., California, Florida, Illinois) (Achman and Chollet, 2001). In general, applicants for coverage through a high-risk pool must demonstrate evidence of ineligibility for coverage at a reasonable charge. States typically cap premium rates at 125 to 200 percent of standard market rates (Achman and Chollet, 2001).

States finance high-risk pools through surcharges on health insurance premiums, from tobacco taxes, general funds, or some combination of these sources. However, only limited revenues are available through state premium taxes, because the Employee Retirement Income Security Act of 1974 (ERISA) exempts self-insured plans from paying them (Achman and Chollet, 2001). A new federal program to help states create high-risk pools was announced in November 2002 (DHHS press release, 2002). Grants of up to $1 million are available to 27 states and the District of Columbia through the Centers for Medicare and Medicaid Services. In addition, another $80 million was appropriated over two years to offset a portion of losses incurred by states from operating high-risk pools.

Some states, in addition to, or instead of, reliance on high-risk pools, regulate the individual market to require guaranteed issue (i.e., a requirement to sell to all applicants irregardless of their medical history). States may also restrict the extent to which premium rates can vary based on health status and/or age. According to a 2001 report, 13 states required insurers to guarantee issue or hold open-enrollment periods, 16 states limited the extent to which insurers could vary rates overall, and 8 states prohibited insurers from considering health status in setting rates (Achman and Chollet, 2001). Four states (Arizona, Delaware, Georgia, and North Carolina) had no specific regulation of the individual insurance market designed to improve either access to or affordability of coverage for people with significant health problems (Achman and Chollet, 2001).

Federal Health Insurance and Disability Programs

Childhood cancer survivors may benefit from various federal health insurance and disability programs, most of which are designed to support those from families with low incomes.

Medicaid and S-Chip

Medicaid is a joint federal/state insurance program for low income and certain disabled individuals. As of 2000, an estimated 26 percent of children and young adults under age 21 were Medicaid beneficiaries (*www.hcfa.gov/medicaid/msis/2082-9.htm*, accessed March 28, 2002). Coverage of uninsured children has been improved through implementation of the State Children's Health Insurance Program (S-CHIP). By fiscal year (FY) 2001, 4.6 million children had ever been enrolled in S-CHIP, many of them through expansions of Medicaid (Centers for Medicare and Medicaid Services, 2002). Medicaid is the single largest source of health care financing for people with disabilities, and covers nearly 7 million people under age 65 with disabilities. However, Medicaid covers only the low-income severely disabled population, leaving significant coverage gaps for other people with disabilities. Most disabled individuals who are Medicaid beneficiaries become eligible through the Supplemental Security Income (SSI) cash assistance program (see below).

The Medicaid program has evolved in recent years from a largely fee-for-service payment system to capitated arrangements. Estimates are that more than half (54 percent) of children and one in four disabled beneficiaries covered by Medicaid are in managed care plans (*www.hcfa.gov/medicaid/msis/2082-9.htm*, accessed March 28, 2002; Kaiser Commission on Medicaid and the Uninsured, 2001).

Under Medicaid's fee-for service arrangements, children with chronic or disabling conditions generally were able to receive specialty care through tertiary care centers and specialty clinics, and from specialty providers (Fox and McManus, 1998). Fully capitated managed care plans may control the use of specialists, especially those outside of their plans' networks. Recommendations for improving state Medicaid contracts and plan practices for children with special needs include (Fox and McManus, 1998):

- clarifying the specificity of pediatric benefits,
- defining appropriate pediatric provider capacity requirements,
- developing a medical necessity standard specific to children,
- identifying pediatric quality-of-care measures,
- setting appropriate pediatric capitation rates, and
- creating incentives for high-quality pediatric care.

Of special interest to survivors of childhood cancer are services provided under Medicaid's Early and Periodic Screening, Diagnosis and Treatment (EPSDT). The scope of services provided under EPSDT is dictated by federal statue and includes "diagnostic, screening, preventive, and rehabilitative services, including medical or remedial services recommended for the maximum reduction of physical or mental disability and restoration of an individual to the best possible functional level (in facility, home, or other setting)" (*http://www.healthlaw.org/pubs/19990323epsdtfact.html*, accessed March 15, 2003). In practice, several barriers to EPSDT have limited the use of services, for example, a shortage of providers participating in the Medicaid program, beneficiaries not being informed of the program and its benefits, and issues related to cost.

State Medicaid programs, while providing a great deal of support, vary by state in terms of coverage and spending, the latter reflecting different provider payment rates, utilization, and other factors.

Supplemental Security Income (SSI)

The Supplemental Security Income program was enacted in 1972 to replace state-run benefit programs for adults who were disabled or over age 65. At the same time, coverage was extended so children with disabilities could quality for federal disability benefits. Eligible children must have evidence of marked and severe functional limitations and their condition must have lasted or be expected to last at least 12 months or be expected to result in the child's death (*www.ssa.gov/pubs/10026.html*, accessed March 15, 2003). Once eligible, disability is redetermined at least every three years. By December 2001, there were an estimated 52,000 individuals under age 65 receiving SSI benefits because of a diagnosis of cancer, 22 percent of them under age 21 (Figure 7.1) (Social Security Bulletin, 2002). SSI is an income support program and as of December 2000, the average monthly SSI payment to families with eligible children was $447 (payment depends on income, and some states provide supplemental payments) (Social Security Administration, 2001). Children under age 18 who qualify for SSI because they are disabled and have low family incomes and limited assets are also eligible for coverage under Medicaid in most states. In some states, children who are eligible for SSI because of their impair-

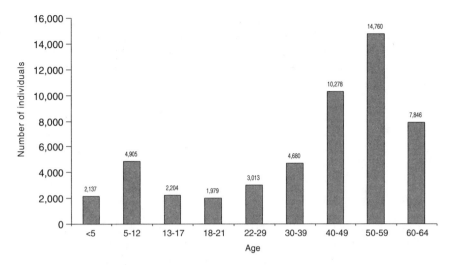

FIGURE 7.1 Number of SSI recipients eligible because of a cancer diagnosis, by age.
SOURCE: Social Security Bulletin, 2002.

ments, but whose families have incomes too high for financial eligibility, can apply for a "Katie Beckett waiver" to allow Medicaid to pay for home and community-based care instead of care in an institution.

Medicare Disability Program

In 1972, Medicare eligibility expanded to include certain disabled individuals under the age of 65. Nonelderly individuals who have received Social Security Disability Insurance (SSDI) payments for 24 months are eligible, but must wait 5 months before receiving disability insurance benefits (they, in effect, must be disabled for 29 months). To be eligible for SSDI, individuals must have limited income and resources and a physical or mental impairment that keeps a person from performing any "substantial" work and is expected to last 12 months or result in death (Social Security Administration, 2002). Individuals diagnosed with end-stage renal disease (ESRD) are also eligible for Medicare regardless of age and financial status. Some adult childhood cancer survivors under age 65 could be eligible for Medicare if they qualified for SSDI or had ESRD. SSDI is an insurance program that provides payments to persons with disabilities based on their having been covered previously under the Social Security program, for example, through their employer. The SSI program is a means-tested income assistance program for disabled, blind, and aged persons who have limited income and resources regardless of their prior participation in the labor force. The definition of disability and the process of determining disability are the same for both programs (Institute of Medicine, 2002).

By 2000, more than 5 million people under age 65 with disabilities or ESRD were enrolled in Medicare (Department of Health and Human Services, 2000). As of 2000, 142,000 individuals under age 65 were receiving SSDI payments because of cancer (of these, 136,000 were disabled workers and 1,700 were individuals disabled as children) (Social Security Bulletin, 2001). Only individuals receiving SSDI benefits for two years would be eligible for Medicare.

Title V Programs

Every state and the District of Columbia has a Title V[2] Program for Children with Special Health Care Needs (CSHCN) that is funded, in part, through the federal Title V Maternal and Child Health Block Grant and provides health and support services to children with special needs and their families (*http://www.mchb.hrsa.gov/programs/default.htm*, assessed March 26, 2003). From the program's inception through the mid 1970s, most of the state programs funded through Title V were called Crippled Children's Services (CCS) Programs and focused their efforts on children with orthopedic problems. In the late 1970s Congress funded state CCS programs to provide case management and care coordination services to children under the age of 16 who received benefits from the SSI program (Schulzinger, 1999). As a result of this expansion, more children with chronic illnesses, developmental disabilities, sensory impairments, and other special health needs were being served and the name of the program was changed to State Programs for Children with Special Health Care Needs (CSHCN). In 1989, Congress amended Title V and required that state CSHCN programs "provide and promote family-centered, community-based, coordinated care (including care coordination services . . .) and to facilitate the development of community-based systems of services for such children and their families." State programs now provide training, finance community support organizations, and promote policies to further coordination and communication. CSHCN programs also provide rehabilitation services to children under age 16 who are receiving SSI, when Medicaid does not pay for those services.

---

[2] Title V refers to the Title of the Social Security Act, enacted in 1935, to provide funds to states to develop and operate public health care programs for certain children with special health care needs as well as to establish other programs to promote the health of low income mothers and children (*http://www.mchb.hrsa.gov/programs/default.htm*, accessed March 26, 2003)

The federal legislation gives states flexibility to use their Title V funds to design and implement direct care programs and services that are responsive to the needs in their state. State programs have different financial and medical criteria and provide different kinds of health care and related services. According to published eligibility criteria for Title V programs, 8 states specifically include cancer as a qualifying condition, and 8 states specifically exclude cancer as a qualifying condition. In the 8 states for which cancer is excluded, some have eligibility criteria that could make services available to cancer survivors with late effects (e.g., cardiac, neurologic, and developmental delay) (Health Resources and Services Administration, 2000). In 1998, 517,000 children were served at a cost of $1.8 billion (an average of $3,557 per child) (Health Resources and Services Administration, 2000) (Table 7.1).

The Maternal and Child Health Bureau and its key partners, including provider and consumer groups, have identified six core desirable outcomes for measurement as part of the Healthy People 2010 initiative (Health Resources and Services Administration, 2001):

1. All children with special health care needs will receive coordinated ongoing comprehensive care within a medical home.

2. All families of children with special health care needs will have adequate private and/or public insurance to pay for the services they need.

3. All children will be screened early and continuously for special health care needs.

4. Families of children with special health care needs will partner in decision making at all levels and will be satisfied with the services they receive.

5. Community-based service systems will be organized so families can use them easily.

6. All youth with special health care needs will receive the services necessary to make transitions to all aspects of adult life, including adult health care, work, and independence.

A national communication strategy, efforts at capacity building, setting standards, and establishing accountability systems are among the activities planned to implement these goals (Health Resources and Services Administration, 2001).

Issues Related to Managed Care

Many children receive care through a managed care plan offered by either a private insurer, Medicaid, or S-CHIP plans. Improved access to primary care and coordination of care are potential benefits of managed

TABLE 7.1 Children with Special Health Care Needs Served in FY 1998 by Each State and the Related Total and Per Child Expenditures Under the Title V Federal-State Block Grants

State	Children with Special Health Care Needs Under Title V Federal-State Block Grants		
	Number of Children Served	Expenditures FY 1998 (million)	Average Expenditure per Child Served FY 1998 (million)
Alabama	22,300	$16.9	$758
Alaska	2,458	5.1	2,075
Arizona	15,349	6.8	443
Arkansas	15,159	4.7	310
California	133,007	912.8	6,862
Colorado	8,272	6.5	786
Connecticut	5,284	3.3	625
Delaware	2,732	0.5	183
District of Columbia	892	1.9	2,130
Florida	47,581	102.8	2,161
Georgia	15,105	30.7	2,032
Hawaii	8,567	7.6	887
Idaho	2,276	2.1	923
Illinois	24,626	24.5	995
Indiana	9,314	19.3	2,072
Iowa	5,430	4.3	792
Kansas	10,972	3.2	292
Kentucky	16,060	9.1	567
Louisiana	8,466	9.5	1,122
Maine	2,247	3.4	1,513
Maryland	14,125	7.4	524
Massachusetts	22,988	29.3	1,275
Michigan	27,550	34.1	1,238
Minnesota	7,309	7.2	985
Mississippi	6,249	7.9	1,264
Missouri	5,647	7.0	1,240

care plans. There are, however, potential disadvantages within managed care plans for children with special health care needs who need specialized complex care. A work group convened by the federal Maternal and Child Health Bureau in 2000 reviewed managed care issues of concern to children with special health care needs. Problems in three areas were identified that are of relevance to childhood cancer survivors: capacity and expertise in managed care organizations, access to specialized pediatric services, and reimbursement (McManus et al., 2000) (Box 7.1).

Recommended approaches that can be adopted by managed care plans

TABLE 7.1 Continued

| State | Children with Special Health Care Needs Under Title V Federal-State Block Grants | | |
	Number of Children Served	Expenditures FY 1998 (million)	Average Expenditure per Child Served FY 1998 (million)
Montana	1,379	1.5	1,088
Nebraska	4,097	2.0	488
Nevada	7,148	1.6	224
New Hampshire	4,238	3.1	732
New Jersey	67,839	8.6	127
New Mexico	12,256	4.6	375
New York	60,763	328.4	5,404
North Carolina	64,787	54.7	844
North Dakota	1,799	1.1	612
Ohio	31,572	32.7	1,036
Oklahoma	16,727	3.9	233
Oregon	7,748	3.3	426
Pennsylvania	33,593	11.5	342
Rhode Island	3,700	4.2	1,135
South Carolina	13,589	22.1	1,626
South Dakota	5,576	1.3	233
Tennessee	4,695	6.5	1,385
Texas	26,848	33.0	1,229
Utah	4,320	9.5	2,199
Vermont	3,624	1.5	414
Virginia	11,160	11.8	1,057
Washington	9,165	5.0	546
West Virginia	5,126	12.7	2,478
Wisconsin	1,896	5.5	2,901
Wyoming	3,137	2.3	733
TOTAL	517,423	1840.2	3557

SOURCE: Health Resources and Services Administration, 2000.

to improve care for children with special health care needs include (Fox and McManus, 1998):

- ensuring that assigned primary care providers have appropriate training and experience,
- offering support systems for primary care practices,
- providing specialty consultation for primary care providers,
- establishing arrangements for the comanagement of primary and specialty pediatric services,

---

Box 7.1
Managed Care Issues of Concern to Children with Special Health Care Needs

Capacity and expertise in managed care organizations

• Shortages in certain pediatric medical and surgical subspecialists (e.g., neurologists, psychiatrists, and other mental health care providers) are being reported in certain parts of the United States.
• Comprehensive pediatric provider networks are not consistently available, making specialty referrals problematic. Oftentimes children with chronic conditions are referred to adult specialists who have limited experience and training in the care of childhood conditions.
• Many children with chronic conditions have difficulty obtaining medical homes because of the complexities of their care and the lack of adequate financial compensation.
• Few multidisciplinary practice arrangements exist to serve children with complex conditions.
• Case management in managed care organizations is often difficult to access and is generally limited to only high-cost children. These services focus on benefit management, not care coordination.
• Many families are assuming too much nursing care responsibility for their children with serious medical conditions.

Access to specialized pediatric services

• There is enormous variation in utilization review and prior authorization criteria among managed care organizations, making it very burdensome for pediatricians and family physicians who contract with multiple plans and need approval for physician and other specialized services.

• arranging for comprehensive care coordination,
• establishing flexible service authorization policies,
• implementing provider profiling systems that adjust for pediatric case mix,
• creating financial incentives for serving children with special needs, and
• encouraging family involvement in plan operations.

LIFE INSURANCE

Obtaining life insurance coverage is difficult for survivors of childhood cancer largely because they have not established their careers and families at the time of their cancer diagnosis. They do not face financial and life planning issues until several years after their cancer treatment. Since life insurance plans are based on an actuarial risk of death (or survival), the

- Managed care plans often apply restrictive medical necessity criteria, limiting access to certain services (e.g., medication, therapies) or limiting the duration of treatment.
- Utilization management staff and case managers in managed care organizations often have limited knowledge about chronic childhood conditions.
- Communication between medical, behavioral, and educational service systems is oftentimes limited and administratively complex

Reimbursement

- Pediatricians serving a disproportionate number of children with chronic conditions are experiencing serious financial difficulties because of the unreimbursed time and services they provide.
- Accepting full-risk capitation for children with chronic conditions is problematic since there are no reliable health risk adjusters for children.
- Reimbursement rates for all pediatric services are much lower than reimbursement rates for adult services
- Managed care organizations and other insurers often fail to reimburse certain Current procedural Terminology (CPT) codes that are needed for the treatment of chronic childhood conditions. These include, but are not limited to prolonged physician service without direct patient contact (99358, 99359); team conferences (99361, 99362); telephone calls (99371-99373); care plan oversight services (99374-99380); preventive medicine, individual counseling (99401-99404); and preventive medicine, group counseling (99411, 99412).
- Few insurers or managed care plans reimburse on the basis of resource-based relative value scale (RBRVS).

SOURCE: McManus et al., 2000.

cancer history is often taken into account because it increases the potential risk of death at an earlier age. Some life insurance companies will not insure cancer survivors, and others will charge very high premiums. Group life insurance (through employment) is a possible solution, since a health history is not usually required for such plans.

SUMMARY AND CONCLUSIONS

Since the early 1990s, significant progress has been made in improving the employment opportunities of cancer survivors. With the recent passage of federal laws such as the Americans with Disabilities Act and the Family and Medical Leave Act, as well as the expansion of many state laws, cancer survivors have gained new legal rights and remedies. Additionally, the rise of cancer survivorship advocacy has helped dispel the myths that fuel survivors' employment problems.

Providing better information to survivors regarding employment rights can lessen the effects of cancer on employment opportunities. From the time of diagnosis, all working-aged (or near working-age) survivors should receive from their cancer center and/or oncologist information about their legal rights, including information about how to avoid employment problems and how to respond to employment discrimination. Additionally, everyone who provides psychosocial support (such as oncology nurses, social workers, therapists, counselors, and peer support organizations) should be familiar with cancer survivors' rights. These health care professionals often are survivors' most important advocates in confronting the psychosocial consequences of cancer. Health care providers can further help their patients avoid job problems by educating employers about their patients' prognoses, abilities, and limitations.

The legal community should become more aware of how current laws apply to cancer survivors' employment rights. Legal education programs to teach attorneys, state and federal enforcement agencies, and the judiciary how laws such as the ADA and FMLA apply to cancer-based discrimination could improve representation and formulation of legal judgments. Incidences of employment discrimination will probably decrease if more survivors prevail with their claims.

An expansion of educational and direct services programs offered by cancer survivor advocacy organizations might also reduce and ultimately prevent employment discrimination. These programs could include attorney referral programs, personal advocacy assistance, workplace counseling to teach employers about the abilities and needs of cancer survivors to mitigate discrimination and to encourage the development of reasonable accommodations, and public educational materials and programs. Any service program must be able to meet the needs of minority populations that may have language and/or cultural barriers, in addition to their cancer history.

The goal of any health insurance reform should be to ensure that all Americans, regardless of medical history or employment status, have access to affordable, quality medical care. Broad-based national health insurance reform is unlikely to take place in the near future. Instead, cancer survivors' best hope for significant insurance reform rests with federal and state legislation that targets specific issues. Because federal legislation generally covers only federal programs, such as Medicare and Medicaid, many insurance reforms must be addressed at the state level. In some cases, states could, for example, expand access to health insurance through increased support of state high-risk insurance pools. Health insurance reforms to improve patient protections must be considered carefully because when reforms increase the costs of insurance products, reforms can have the unintended consequence of higher rates of uninsurance

Medicaid and Medicare are federally supported programs that provide health insurance to at least some cancer survivors, by virtue of either low income and limited assets or disability. Cancer survivors, if disabled and with limited means, may receive cash assistance or income support through the SSI and SSDI programs. Eligibility for these programs may open the door to health insurance coverage through the Medicaid or Medicare programs. Other state-based programs such as the Title V Children with Special Health Needs programs can provide services such as assistance with health care and rehabilitation, care coordination, and case management. State-based demonstration projects supported through HRSA's Special Projects of Regional and National Significance (SPRANS) and Community Integrated Service Systems (CISS) grants may offer opportunities to learn more about effective health service delivery strategies of relevance to childhood cancer survivors (see description of these grants in Chapter 8).

REFERENCES

Achman L, Chollet D. 2001. Insuring the Uninsurable: An Overview of State High-Risk Health Insurance Pools. Mathematica Policy Research, Inc. Princeton NJ (*http://www.mathematica-mpr.com/3rdlevel/uninsurablehot.htm*, last accessed March 21, 2003).

Burton L, Jones J. 1982. *The Incidence of Insurance Barriers and Employment Discrimination Among Californians With Cancer Health History in 1983.* Oakland, CA: California Division of the American Cancer Society.

Centers for Medicare and Medicaid Services. 2002. *State Children's Health Insurance Program: Fiscal Year 2001 Annual Enrollment Report.* Washington, DC: U.S. DHHS.

Crothers, H.M. 1986. *Employment Problems of Cancer Survivors: Local Program and Local Solutions, Proceedings of the Workshop on Employment Insurance and the Patient With Cancer.* Atlanta, GA: American Cancer Society.

Department of Health and Human Services, HCFA. 2000. *Medicare 2000: 35 Years of Improving Americans' Health and Security.* Washington, DC.

Department of Health and Human Services, CMS. 2002. HHS to Help States Create High-Risk Pools to Increase Access to Health Coverage. Press release, November 26, 2002. (*www.hhs.gov/news/press/2002pres/20021126a.html*, last accessed January 31, 2003).

Ferrell BR, Hassey Dow K. 1997. Quality of life among long-term cancer survivors. *Oncology (Huntingt)* 11(4):565-8, 571; discussion 572, 575-6.

Fobair P, Hoppe RT, Bloom J, Cox R, Varghese A, Spiegel D. 1986. Psychosocial problems among survivors of Hodgkin's disease. *J Clin Oncol* 4(5):805-14.

Fox HB, McManus MA. 1998. Improving state Medicaid contracts and plan practices for children with special needs. *Future Child* 8(2):105-18.

Fox HB, McManus MA. 2001. A national study of commercial health insurance and Medicaid definitions of medical necessity: what do they mean for children? *Ambul Pediatr* 1(1):16-22.

Green DM, Zevon MA, Hall B. 1991. Achievement of life goals by adult survivors of modern treatment for childhood cancer. *Cancer* 67(1):206-13.

Hays DM. 1993. Adult survivors of childhood cancer. Employment and insurance issues in different age groups. *Cancer* 71(10 Suppl):3306-9.

Hays DM, Landsverk J, Sallan SE, Hewett KD, Patenaude AF, Schoonover D, Zilber SL, Ruccione K, Siegel SE. 1992. Educational, occupational, and insurance status of childhood cancer survivors in their fourth and fifth decades of life. *J Clin Oncol* 10(9):1397-406.

Health Resources and Services Administration. 2000. *Title V: A Snapshot of Maternal and Child Health, 2000.* Rockville, MD: Health Resources and Services Administration.

Health Resources and Services Administration. 2001. *Achieving Success for All Children and Youth With Speical Health Care Needs: A 10-Year Action Plan to Accompany Healthy People 2010.* Washington, DC: US DHHS.

Hoffman B, eds. 1996. *A Cancer Survivors' Almanac: Charting Your Journey.* National Coalition for Cancer Survivorship (U.S.). Minneapolis, MN: Chronimed Publishing.

Hoffman B. 1999. Cancer survivors' employment and insurance rights: a primer for oncologists. *Oncology (Huntingt)* 13(6):841-6; discussion 846, 849, 852.

Hoffman B. 2000. *Between a Disability and a Hard Place: The Cancer Survivors' Catch-22 of Proving Disability Status Under the Americans With Disabilities Act.* Baltimore, MD: Maryland Law Review .

Hoffman B. 2002a. Policy Recommendations to Address the Employment and Insurance Concerns of Cancer Survivors (IOM commissioned background paper). (www.nas.edu).

Institute of Medicine. 2002. *The Dynamics of Disability: Measuring and Monitoring Disability for Social Security Programs.* Washington DC: National Academy Press.

Kaiser Commission on Medicaid and the Uninsured. 2001. *Medicaid's Role for the Disabled Population Under Age 65 .* Washington, DC: The Henry J. Kaiser Family Foundation.

Koocher G, O'Malley J. 1982. *The Damocles Syndrome.* McGraw Hill: New York.

Kornblith AB, Herndon JE 2nd, Zuckerman E, Cella DF, Cherin E, Wolchok S, Weiss RB, Diehl LF, Henderson E, Cooper MR, Schiffer C, Canellos GP, Mayer RJ, Silver RT, Schilling A, Peterson BA, Greenberg D, Holland JC. 1998. Comparison of psychosocial adaptation of advanced stage Hodgkin's disease and acute leukemia survivors. Cancer and Leukemia Group B. *Ann Oncol* 9(3):297-306.

McManus M, Fox H, Newacheck P. 2000. *Report From an Expert Working Group: Pediatric Provider Networks for Children With Special Needs in the Current Health Insurance Market.* Washington DC: HRSA, U.S. DHHS.

Monaco GP, Fiduccia D, Smith G. 1997. Legal and societal issues facing survivors of childhood cancer. *Pediatr Clin North Am* 44(4):1043-58.

Pang PW, Friedman DL, Whitton J, Weiss NS, Mertens A, Robison L. 2002. Employment Status of Adult Survivors of Pediatric Cancers: A Report from the Childhood Cancer Survivors Study (CCSS). Poster Presentation. Cancer Survivorship: Resilience Across the Lifespan. National Cancer Institute, Washington, DC. June 2-4.

President's Cancer Panel NCI. 2001. Voices of a Broken System: Real People, Real Problems. *Report of the Chairman, 2000-2001.* Bethesda, MD: National Cancer Institute.

Schulzinger R. Institute for Child Health Policy. 1999. *State Title V Rehabilitation Services: The Federal Law and How States Implement It.* Gainesville, FL.

Social Security Administration. 2001. *Children Receiving SSI December 2000.* Baltimore, MD: Social Security Administration, Office of Policy, Office of Research, Evaluation, and Statistics, Division of SSI Statistics and Analysis.

Social Security Administration. 2002. *A Desktop Guide to SSI Eligibility Requirements.* Baltimore, MD: Social Security Administration.

Social Security Bulletin. 2001. *Annual Statistical Supplement.* Baltimore, MD: Social Security Administration.

Social Security Bulletin. 2002. *SSI Annual Statistical Report.* Baltimore, MD: Social Security Administration.

Teta MJ, Del Po MC, Kasl SV, Meigs JW, Myers MH, Mulvihill JJ. 1986. Psychosocial consequences of childhood and adolescent cancer survival. *J Chronic Dis* 39(9):751-9.

Vann JC, Biddle AK, Daeschner CW, Chaffee S, Gold SH. 1995. Health insurance access to young adult survivors of childhood cancer in North Carolina. *Med Pediatr Oncol* 25(5):389-95.

Wasserman AL, Thompson EI, Wilimas JA, Fairclough DL. 1987. The Psychological Status of Survivors of Childhood/Adolescent Hodgkin's Disease. *American Journal of Diseases of Children* 141(6):626-31.

Weiner SL, McCabe MS, Smith GP, Monaco GP, Fiduccia D. 2002. Pediatric Cancer: Advocacy Insurance, Education, and Employment. Pizzo PA, Poplack DG, (eds). *Principles and Practice of Pediatric Oncology.* Philadelphia: Lippincott Williams and Wilkins. Pp. 1512-1526.

White PH. 2002. Access to health care: health insurance considerations for young adults with special health care needs/disabilities. Pediatrics 110(6 Pt 2):1328-35.

Working Woman/Amgen. 1996. *Cancer in the Workplace Survey.* Working Woman/ Amgen.

Yankelovich CS. 1992. *Cerenex Survey on Cancer Patients in the Workplace: Breaking Down Discrimination Barriers.* Unpublished.

8

Research Issues

The first attempts to ascertain the prevalence of late effects of childhood cancer were made in the mid 1970s by Anna Meadows and her colleagues at the Children's Hospital of Philadelphia (Meadows and D'Angio, 1974; Meadows et al., 1975; Meadows and Evans, 1976). Nearly three decades later, much remains to be known. This chapter reviews types of research of relevance to cancer survivorship, describes major ongoing survivorship research initiatives, and summarizes the state of survivorship research and levels of support. The chapter concludes with a listing of prioritized areas of research identified by the Board.

SURVIVORSHIP RESEARCH

Research of relevance to survivors of cancer generally aims to: (1) identify late effects and their implications for health and well-being; (2) modify and improve cancer treatment to minimize late effects; and (3) develop post-treatment interventions to reduce the consequences of late effects for individuals and their families. Research to date has focused primarily in the first two areas. There has been limited research on interventions to prevent late effects among high-risk individuals or on strategies to ameliorate the consequences of late effects among individuals who have developed them. Also lacking are studies of survivors and their families regarding the psychosocial burden and economic costs associated with late effects.

Research to Identify Late Effects and Their Implications

Most of what has been learned about the late effects of cancer treatment has been the result of longitudinal or cross-sectional studies of survivors treated according to standard protocols within single institutions. These investigations have provided important insights into the frequency and potential risk factors for late effects occurring at relatively high frequency. Such studies have, for example, helped to identify impaired fertility following alkylating agent treatments, hearing impairment following cisplatin-based chemotherapy regimens, and restrictive lung disease following pulmonary radiation. Because these studies were conducted in a single institution, included few subjects, and involved treatment that did not vary markedly across subjects, estimates of risk associated with variations in treatment could usually not be well quantified.

Some studies of long-term survivors have been carried out within established pediatric cooperative groups (e.g., Children's Cancer Group [CCG], Pediatric Oncology Group [POG], National Wilms Tumor Study Group [NWTSG], Intergroup Rhabdomyosascoma Study Group [IRSG]).[1] The primary objective of these groups is to conduct therapeutic clinical trials; and while questions of health-related outcomes are of interest, the resources necessary to support such studies have generally not been available. The potential to conduct research on late effects in these settings is substantial because as many as 50 to 60 percent of U.S. children with cancer are treated at Children's Oncology Group (COG) member institutions (Shochat et al., 2001). A Late Effects Committee established in the mid 1980s promotes and facilitates research on adverse health-related outcomes after childhood cancer (Bhatia, 2002). Research efforts in this area have, however, been limited (Box 8.1). Some of the early findings on cognitive late effects among children with leukemia emerged from follow-up studies of children enrolled in clinical trials of the Cancer and Leukemia Group B Cooperative Group (CALGB). Investigators of the National Wilms' Tumor Study Group (NWTSG) were instrumental in recognizing the late effects of therapies among survivors of Wilms' tumor and adjusting treatment (e.g., omission of radiotherapy) in an effort to avoid these late side effects.

COG has plans for a long- term follow-up center to provide a cost-effective mechanism for tracking and maintaining contact with patients and their families and for collecting long-term data on health and health-related quality of life. This system complements a web-based remote data entry

---

[1]The National Cancer Institute-sponsored pediatric cooperative groups, now merged into the Children's Oncology Group, are also discussed in Chapter 5.

Box 8.1
Past, Current, and Planned Research Activities of
COG's Late Effects Committee

Past studies: 8 publications on second malignant neoplasms, neuropsychological, cardiac and other health-related outcomes (cancers studied included acute lymphoblastic leukemia (ALL), Wilms tumor, Rhabdomyosarcoma, osteosarcoma, Ewing's sarcoma)

Current studies:

• Validation of a Quality of Life (QOL) tool for cancer survivors
• QOL and neuropsychological impairment after intracranial gliomas
• QOL after acute myelogenous leukemia (AML)
• QOL after neuroblastoma
• National Wilms Tumor Study Late Effects study
• Reproductive endocrine function after osteosarcoma
• Second malignant neoplasms after childhood cancer
• Clinical biological predictors of therapy related acute myeloidleukemia/myelodysplasia (t-AML/MDS).

Proposed studies:

• Neurocognitive and QOL assessment
• Gene-environment interaction
• Late mortality after childhood cancer

SOURCE: Bhatia, 2002.

system for all patients entering COG studies at member institutions. Member institutions report each individual diagnosed with cancer who is seen at the institutions to the COG Research Data Center Registry of New Malignancies in Children and Adolescents (Children's Oncology Group, 2001). Patient responses to therapy are centrally collected, monitored, and analyzed. With these mechanisms in place, patients treated within COG institutions could potentially be followed prospectively and their outcomes linked to their primary treatments.

For research encompassing extended intervals from the original cancer diagnosis (e.g., two or more decades), well-designed cohort studies are needed. Organized consortia have been able to successfully address selected topics relating to childhood cancer survivorship. The Late Effects Study Group (LESG), an international consortium of institutions, has provided important insights into the risk of second malignancies, particularly among Hodgkin's disease survivors (Bhatia et al., 1996).

Childhood Cancer Survivor Study (CCSS)

The Childhood Cancer Survivor Study (CCSS) is a large, National Cancer Institute-sponsored, multi-institutional initiative to organize a cohort of survivors for long-term follow-up. Included in the cohort are 20,276 childhood cancer survivors diagnosed between 1970 and 1986 who have survived 5 or more years after treatment (Robison et al., 2002); *http://www.cancer.umn. edu/ltfu*, accessed March 25, 2002). The study also includes approximately 3,500 siblings of survivors, who serve as control subjects for the study. The CCSS cohort has been assembled through the efforts of 27 participating centers in the United States and Canada and is coordinated by investigators at the University of Minnesota. Initiated in 1993, the study was recently funded by the National Cancer Institute for continuation through 2004.

Selected demographic and cancer-related characteristics of the CCSS cohort are shown in Table 8.1.

To date, baseline information has been collected, including demographic data and treatment history of study participants as well as data regarding the occurrence of cancer and certain hereditary conditions in their first-degree relatives. In addition to completing the baseline questionnaire, survivors agreed to release medical records of their cancer treatment. Participating centers have provided detailed abstracts of treatment records for all consenting survivors enrolled in the cohort from their site. Treatment information includes cumulative dose-specific exposure to chemotherapy, surgical procedures, and radiation therapy. Follow-up data (information from medical charts and self-reported information on health status and behaviors) has been collected from participants, and investigators have begun collecting biologic materials, including tumor specimens from participants who develop subsequent cancers, buccal (cheek) cells from all participants—including siblings—as a source of genomic DNA, and peripheral blood samples from a subset of survivors and sibling controls to establish cell lines as a source of genomic DNA and RNA. These materials will be used to evaluate the role of genetics in the occurrence of cancer and long-term adverse outcomes among survivors.

A likely outcome of a large cohort study such as the CCSS is the early identification of emerging or changing patterns of late effects. With the increasing age of the population of childhood cancer survivors, it is anticipated that new adverse health-related outcomes are likely to emerge. With continued surveillance, these new and/or unexpected events can be ascertained and characterized. Cohorts like CCSS can provide an early warning system for the emergence of unrecognized late effects of treatment. An example is the relatively recent appreciation of the magnitude of excess risk for breast cancer in patients treated for Hodgkin's disease during child-

TABLE 8.1 Characteristics of the CCSS Participants
(n = 14,054)

Characteristic	Percent
Sex	
Male	54
Female	46
Race	
White	87
Black	2
Hispanic	5
Asian/Pacific Islander	1
Other	5
Diagnosis	
Leukemia	34
Brain/CNS	13
Hodgkin's	14
Non-Hodgkin's	7
Kidney	9
Neuroblastoma	7
Soft-tissue sarcoma	9
Bone	8
Age at diagnosis	
<1 year	7
1 to 3 years	25
4 to 7 years	22
8 to 10 years	11
11 to 14 years	17
15 to 20 years	18
Age at entry on CCSS	
<20 years	32
20 to 29 years	42
30 to 39 years	22
40+ years	3

SOURCE: Robinson et al., 2002.

hood. This observed association was identified through the LESG cohort of Hodgkin's disease survivors. Adverse events recognized in smaller studies can be confirmed and further defined in existing cohort studies and the information used to develop new protocols that seek to minimize such complications. Some late effects may be observed among long-term survivors following exposures to therapies that are no longer in use. Studies of more recent cohorts exposed to newer treatments are needed to ascertain declines in treatment-related late effects and the emergence of new late effects.

Ongoing contact and interaction offers an opportunity to provide survivors with information regarding cancer survivorship, and allows survivors to make their concerns and ideas known.

Current and proposed research based on the CCSS cohort is shown in Box 8.2.

While cohort studies such as the CCSS provide invaluable information pertaining to late effects, such studies are difficult to conduct and have some inherent limitations. The greatest challenge in these studies is enrolling and maintaining a cohort of patients that represents the population of patients eligible for the study. A nonrepresentative cohort could result if only certain patients volunteered for the study, or if patients who did enroll were lost to follow up on the basis of an important study variable. If, for example, patients who entered the study and then became very ill were more difficult to follow up, their absence in the follow-up period could contribute to the failure to associate an exposure during treatment to subsequent morbidity or mortality.

Gathering longitudinal information on children is especially difficult because of the problem of frequent moves. Participants may also be lost to follow-up when they turn age 18 and must provide consent for study participation (prior to that age, parents provide consent). Interest in participating in research may wane among adolescents and young adults. Obtaining medical records regarding care is complicated when children's providers change and when they transition from pediatric to adult providers. Obtaining accurate information regarding treatment-related exposures and health-related outcomes is key to the success of a cohort study, but the inaccessibility and sometimes incomplete nature of medical records can compromise the ability to obtain such information.

Resources can be marshaled to overcome many of the practical difficulties of tracking cohort members and keeping them engaged in the study. A well-conducted cohort study can provide estimates of the prevalence of late effects and the degree of excess risk. It can also provide invaluable information on quality-of-life outcomes such as achievement and progress in school, employment, and use and satisfaction with health care. Such information can help guide program development and the design of interventions.

Research to Modify or Improve Cancer Treatment to Minimize Late Effects

Once late effects have been recognized, clinical trials can be designed to test modifications of treatments that are likely to reduce their occurrence. A clinical trial involving children with localized lymphomas demonstrated that radiation therapy can be safely omitted without jeopardizing high cure rates (Link et al., 1997). More recently, researchers have conducted trials

Box 8.2
Current and Proposed CCSS Analyses

Mortality

- Late mortality in 5-year survivors of childhood cancer

Physical late effects
- Second primary neoplasms following childhood cancer
- Risk factors for secondary solid tumors after Hodgkin's disease
- Second neoplasms of the central nervous system in survivors of childhood cancer
- Second primary neoplasms following childhood leukemia: a report from CCSS
- Pain sequelae in survivors of childhood cancer
- Thyroid disease in survivors of childhood and adolescent Hodgkin's disease
- Cardiac outcomes in survivors of childhood cancer
- Physical disabilities after treatment for childhood cancer

Reproductive consequences
- Cancer in offspring of pediatric cancer survivors
- Pregnancy outcomes after treatment for cancer during childhood and adolescence
- Fertility rates among long-term survivors of Hodgkin's disease diagnosed during childhood

Genetics
- Family history in survivors of pediatric Hodgkin's disease

Psychosocial late effects
- Marriage in survivors of childhood cancer
- Neurological, psychosocial, and risk behavior in survivors of childhood cancer
- Suicide and suicidal ideation among childhood cancer survivors

Behavioral risk factors
- Smoking among childhood cancer survivors
- Participation in and predictors of physical activity among childhood cancer survivors
- Health practice among childhood cancer survivors: Implications for cancer control
- Utilization of special education services among adult survivors
- Confirmatory factor analysis of the Brief Symptoms Inventory depression and anxiety scales in the survivor population

Economic and health care consequences
- Insurance and insurability in the Childhood Cancer Survivor Study cohort
- Barriers to long-term health care for childhood cancer survivors

Methods
- Predicting loss to follow-up and successful tracing in childhood cancer survivors
- The Childhood Cancer Survivor Study: A Collaborative Study

SOURCE: *http://www.cancer.umn.edu/ltfu*, accessed March 25, 2002.

of agents designed to protect normal tissues from the cytotoxic effects of chemotherapy and radiation (amifostine or dexrazoxane [Zinecard®]) to evaluate their promise of fewer adverse effects in survivors of cancer treatment. Another strategy to minimize late effects while maintaining high rates of survival involves tailoring treatments to patients' risk status, and assigning less intense treatment for patients with a lower risk of relapse, with the expectation that this group would have less frequent and severe acute toxicity, fewer and milder late effects, and a better quality of long-term survival. Risk strata are determined using a combination of clinical and biologic prognostic indicators. There are many examples of evaluations of risk-adapted treatments, including those for childhood acute lymphoblastic leukemia (Smith et al., 1996), rhabdomyosarcoma (Raney et al., 2001), and neuroblastoma (Castleberry, 1997). Long-term follow-up is needed as part of these studies to assure safety and efficacy.

Research on Interventions to Reduce the Consequences of Late Effects

Interventional research designed to prevent the emergence of late effects and to reverse or forestall the progression of already-established complications of cancer treatment is less advanced, but urgently needed. Approaches in this area include the use of hormone replacement therapy or chemoprevention for reduction of the risk of second malignant neoplasms among high-risk populations, and after-load reduction therapy with ACE inhibitors such as enalapril in patients with asymptomatic left ventricular dysfunction following anthracycline treatment. Secondary prevention approaches also need to be tested in efforts to forestall or ameliorate late effects. Lifestyle counseling, family interventions to address psychosocial issues, and educational interventions to improve cognitive function are examples of such areas of needed research.

STATUS OF CHILDHOOD SURVIVORSHIP RESEARCH

This section first describes publication trends in childhood cancer survivorship and then summarizes federal and private support for such research.

Publication Trends

The evaluation of trends in research publications is one way to assess the level of activity within a discipline. One resource that can be used to track such studies is the National Library of Medicine's PubMed database, which stores information about individual citations including index terms used to characterize each article (articles are indexed according to a dictionary of medical subject headings called MESH terms). The PubMed data-base includes citations from MedLine, HealthStar, and other bibliographic databases.

There have been few English-language articles on childhood cancer survivorship in recent years; however, the volume of articles appears to have increased somewhat from 1993 to 2001, from 101 to 153 (Figure 8.1). In 2001, these articles accounted for less than 3 percent of all pediatric cancer-related citations indexed in the medical literature (Figure 8.2). While there are relatively few published articles regarding childhood survivorship, they represent a relatively large share of citations on survivorship, nearly a third (31.9 percent) of such citations in 2001 (Figure 8.3). These trends reflect articles written in the English language, but not necessarily by U.S. investigators. Figures 8.1, 8.2, and 8.3 therefore reflect trends in the general medical literature, and not necessarily trends in the United States. These trends must be interpreted with caution because they may reflect changes in the ways in which MESH headings were applied to index the literature rather than real increases in cancer-related research. The term "survivors," the MESH heading used to identify citations, refers to "per-

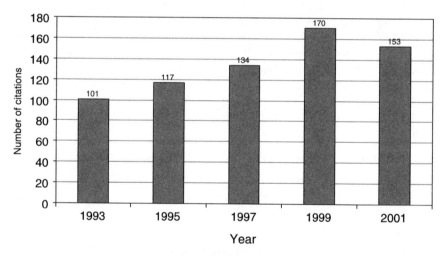

FIGURE 8.1 PubMed citations for childhood cancer survivorship research, 1993-2001.
NOTE: A wildcard allows any ending to follow the base word in replace of the asterisk. For instance, survivors and survivorship would be included in a keyword search of survivor*.
SOURCE: National Library of Medicine's PubMed database.

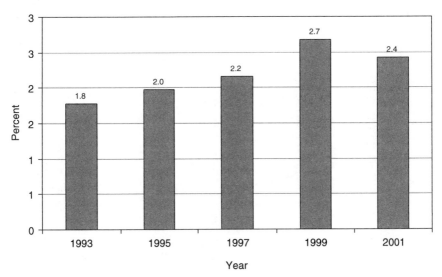

FIGURE 8.2 PubMed citations for childhood cancer survivorship research as a percentage of all pediatric cancer-related citations, 1993-2001. Percentages were calculated as the numbre of childhood cancer survivorship-related citations (as described in Figure 8.1) divided by the total number of citations categorized under the MESH terms "neoplasms" and either "pediatrics" or "child." Only articles published in English are counted.
SOURCE: National Library of Medicine's PubMed database.

sons who have experienced a prolonged survival after serious disease or who continue to live with a usually life-threatening condition as well as family members, significant others, or individuals surviving traumatic life events" (*http://www.ncbi.nlm.nih.gov:80/entrez/meshbrowser.cgi*, accessed March 25, 2002). Both keywords and MESH headings were used to identify citations. There would be an underestimate of survivorship- related citations if the "Survivors" MESH term was not applied by abstractors to the citations or if the title and abstracts of articles varied in their inclusion of keywords (e.g., survivors, survivorship, late effect, long-term effects).

SUPPORT FOR SURVIVORSHIP RESEARCH

A more direct way to assess the status of U.S.-based research on childhood cancer survivors is to describe topics of investigation and levels of research spending. There is no one comprehensive source of information on research support, and as part of its review, the National Cancer Policy Board relied on the following sources:

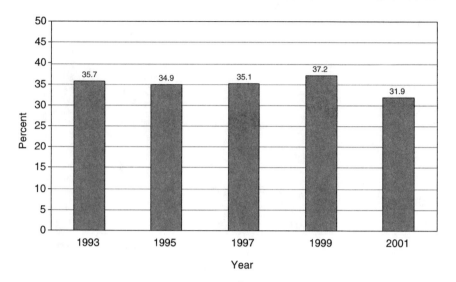

FIGURE 8.3 PubMed citations for childhood cancer survivorship research as a percentage of all cancer survivorship-related research, 1993-2001. Percentages were calculated as the numbre of childhood cancer survivorship-related citations (as described in Figure 8.1) divided by the total number of citations categorized under the MESH terms "neoplasms" and either "pediatrics" or "child." Only articles published in English are counted.

NOTE: A wildcard allows any ending to follow the base word in replace of the asterisk. For instance, survivors and survivorship would be included in a keyword search of survivor*.

SOURCE: National Library of Medicine's PubMed database.

• Listings of research projects in the CRISP (Computer Retrieval of Information on Scientific Projects), a searchable database of federally funded biomedical research projects conducted at universities, hospitals, and other research institutions,[2]

• Review of organizations' web sites,

• Presentations to the Board by agency representatives (e.g., NCI, Office of Cancer Survivorship), and

---

[2] The database, maintained by the Office of Extramural Research at the National Institutes of Health, includes projects funded by the National Institutes of Health (NIH), Substance Abuse and Mental Health Services (SAMHSA), Health Resources and Services Administration (HRSA), Food and Drug Administration (FDA), Centers for Disease Control and Prevention (CDCP), Agency for Health Care Research and Quality (AHRQ), and Office of Assistant Secretary of Health (OASH) (*https://www-commons.cit.nih.gov/crisp/*, accessed March 25, 2002).

• Contacts with organization representatives (e.g., American Cancer Society, Lance Armstrong Foundation, Centers for Disease Control and Prevention).

The Board's review of research support is limited to federal agencies, primarily the National Institutes of Health and selected private organizations and foundations (i.e., American Cancer Society, Lance Armstrong Foundation). Although these organizations are not the only sponsors of research on cancer survivorship, they represent the major funding sources for such research. Excluded from this review is research supported by health plans, insurers, pharmaceutical companies, and other private organizations. Much of the research done in those settings is proprietary.

Federal Research Support

National Cancer Institute

NCI supports research through a variety of mechanisms, including cooperative agreements (referred to as U01 or U19 cooperative agreements), and investigator-initiated grants (referred to as R01 and P01 grants). The largest investment in childhood cancer research is through support of pediatric clinical trials cooperative groups and other research consortia. Each year about 4,000 children enter one of approximately 100 ongoing clinical trials sponsored by NCI (National Cancer Institute, 2002a). And as part of the Childhood Cancer Survivor Study, a cohort of more than 20,000 5-year survivors are being followed. In fiscal year 2001, NCI spent $128 million to support studies of the biology, causes, and effective treatment of pediatric cancer, and to support research on the health status and well-being of children surviving cancer (National Cancer Institute, 2002a). Much of this research is conducted through the following organized pediatric cooperative groups and research consortia (National Cancer Institute, 2002a):

• **Children's Oncology Group** involves 238 member institutions in the conduct of clinical trials for children and adolescents with cancer (see map showing U.S. member institutions in Chapter 5). The group was formed in 2000 to merge the Children's Cancer Group (CCG), Intergroup Rhabdomyosarcoma Study Group (IRSG), National Wilm's Tumor Study Group (NWTSG), and the Pediatric Oncology Group (POG),
• **Pediatric Brain Tumor Consortium** involves nine academic institutions that conduct phase 1 and 2 clinical evaluations of new therapeutic drugs, intrathecal agents, delivery technologies, biological therapies, and radiation treatment strategies in children and young adults (up to age 21) with primary CNS tumors,

• **New Approaches to Neuroblastoma Therapy Consortium** involves eight university and children's hospitals to test promising new therapies for neuroblastoma, and
    • **Childhood Cancer Survivor Study** involves 27 participating centers in the United States and Canada in following a cohort of over 20,000 5-year survivors of childhood cancer (see description above). The study was initiated in 1993 and is funded through 2004.

Office of Cancer Survivorship   The locus of cancer survivorship research at the federal level is the NCI's Office of Cancer Survivorship (OCS), established in 1996 to support research on the physical, psychosocial, and economic consequences of cancer among survivors (of all ages), their families, and caregivers (National Cancer Institute, 1999; National Cancer Institute, 2002b). The OCS supports research related to:

• the identification, prevention, and amelioration of the late effects of cancer and its treatment,
    • follow-up care and surveillance of cancer survivors, and
    • communication to cancer survivors and their families and public education regarding survivorship issues.

OCS awarded its first research grants in 1997, totaling $4 million over 2 years (National Cancer Institute, 1999). In 1998, OCS awarded another $15 million over 5 years. OCS awarded $1 million in 2000 to support supplements to comprehensive cancer centers (P30s) to conduct pilot or exploratory research on issues related to the functioning of family members of survivors. In 2001, using a similar mechanism, OCS awarded an additional $1.06 million to support pilot research on issues faced by minority and underserved cancer survivors. The OCS has also participated in two trans-NIH Requests for Applications (RFAs), which led to funding of a mind-body center in cancer at a cost of $10 million over 5 years, and research on adherence to post-treatment interventions budgeted at $2 million over 4 years. While OCS does not have any initiatives with set-aside funds designated for 2002, the office actively encourages investigators to utilize a number of existing program announcements (PAs). These include s the R03 and R21 Behavioral PAs, the Epidemiologic Cohort PA, and a number of trans-NIH collaborative initiatives (such as those on sleep, palliative care, physical activity), all of which contain language relevant to cancer survivorship research, designed to stimulate and support research (Julia Rowland, NCI Office of Cancer Survivorship, personal communication to Maria Hewitt, June 19, 2002).
    NCI-supported research in childhood survivorship is shown in Box 8.3 along with other NIH-supported survivorship research.

In its budget proposal for Fiscal Year 2004, the NCI has identified cancer survivorship as an "Extraordinary Opportunity for Investment." Extraordinary Opportunities for Investment are identified with formal input from members of the research community, advisory groups, and advocacy organizations and represent areas of discovery that hold promise for making significant progress against all cancers. The budget proposal includes a request for $46 million to support the following six objectives (National Cancer Institute, 2002c):

1. expand research efforts to understand the biological, physical, psychological, and social mechanisms and their interactions, that affect a cancer patient's response to disease, treatment, and recovery,

2. accelerate the pace of intervention research in order to reduce cancer-related chronic and late morbidity and mortality,

3. develop tools to assess the quality-of- life and care of post-treatment cancer survivors and their family members,

4. enhance NCI's capacity to track outcomes for cancer survivors,

5. ensure the development and dissemination of new interventions and best practices, in collaboration with other federal and health- or cancer-related professional and non-profit organizations, and

6. expand the scientific base for understanding the biologic and physiologic mechanisms in the adverse late effects of current and new cancer treatments.

Specific initiatives identified within each of these objectives relate to cancer survivors of all ages, including survivors of childhood cancer. One initiative—the establishment of a separate registry for pediatric cancer survivors seen within the pediatric clinical trials network—is specific to survivors of childhood cancer.

Health Resources and Services Administration

In 1981 Congress authorized a federal set-aside for Special Projects of Regional and National Significance (SPRANS) as part of the MCH Block Grant (Health Resources and Services Administration, 2000b). Fifteen percent of MCH Block Grant funds support research, training, and demonstration programs (Table 8.2).

Several SPRANS-supported projects and projects supported by another set-aside program authorized by Congress in 1989 (Community Integrated Service Systems or CISS) relate to the integration of services for children with special health needs. Some of these programs attempt to facilitate the development of comprehensive systems of care for individuals with complex chronic conditions such as hemophilia, sickle cell disease, and trau-

Box 8.3
Childhood Survivorship Research Supported by the National Institutes of Health (Extramural Grants)

NCI, Office of Cancer Survivorship
1. Late Effects in Wilms' Tumors Survivors and Offspring
2. Cognitive Remediation for Childhood Cancer Survivors
3. Smoking Cessation among Childhood Cancer Survivors
4. Changing Parental Beliefs in Pediatric Oncology
5. Cardiac Risk Factors in Pediatric Cancer Survivors
6. Learning Impairments Among Survivors of Childhood Cancer
7. Quality of Life Following Successful Therapy for AML
8. Premature Menopause in Survivors of Childhood Cancer
9. Steroid Effects in Pediatric ALL Patients
10. Childhood Cancer Survivors: Spiritual Coping and Adjustment

Other NCI
11. Hepatitis C in Childhood Cancer Survivors
12. Stress, Support and Survival—Children at Medical Risk
13. Psychosocial Outcome in Childhood Cancer Survivors
14. Late Effects in Survivors of Stem Cell Transplantation
15. Therapy-related Leukemia: Clinical/Biologic Predictors
16. Detection and Therapy of Residual Leukemia in Children

Other NIH

National Center for Research Resources
17. Bone Density in Survivors of Pediatric Acute Lymphoblastic Leukemia
18. Cardiac Status in Long Term Survivors of Childhood Cancer

TABLE 8.2 Special Projects of Regional and National Significance (SPRANS) Grant Funding Levels, Fiscal Year 2000 (in Millions), by Category of SPRANS Grant

Category	Funding level ($ in millions)
Total	$109.14
• MCH research	8.53
• MCH training	41.83
• Genetic disease testing, counseling, and information dissemination	9.20
• Hemophilia diagnostic and treatment centers	5.35
• Other special projects to improve maternal and child health	44.24

SOURCE: Health Resources and Services Administration, 2000b.

19.   Growth, Adolescent Development and Body Composition in Survivors of CNS Tumors
20.   Body Composition, Growth, Puberty in Survivors of Childhood ALL and NHL

National Institute for Nursing Research
21.   Resilience and Quality of Life in Adolescents with Cancer
22.   Math Intervention for Children with Leukemia

National Institute for Child Health and Human Development
23.   Impact of Leukemia Treatment on the CNS and Development

National Institute for Deafness and Other Communication
24.   Balancing Survival and Ototoxicity in Cisplatin Therapy

National Institute of Mental Health
25.   Maternal Distress, Cognitive Processing and Pediatric Bone Marrow Transplantation

NOTE: This list was compiled using the OCS current research portfolio and the following four searches of the Computer Retrieval of Information on Scientificc Projects (CRISP) database: (1) "pediatric" and "cancer" and "survivors"; (2) "child" and "cancer" and "survivors"; (3) "child" and "cancer" and "late" and "effects;" and 4) "pediatric" and "cancer" and "late" and "effects."

SOURCE: CRISP, accessed on June 6, 2002; OCS, 2002; Julia Rowland, Director, NCI Office of Cancer Survivorship, personal communication to Maria Hewitt, June 20, 2002. *http:// www.crisp.cit.nih.gov/.*

matic brain injury. Individuals with these conditions share some similarities with childhood cancer survivors in terms of their continuing care needs (Table 8.3).

Private Research Support

This section of the report describes the research activities of two private national organizations that support cancer research relevant to survivors of childhood cancer, the American Cancer Society and the Lance Armstrong Foundation. Many other private organizations provide support for education, advocacy, and service programs (e.g., Candlelighters Childhood Cancer Foundation; the Starbright Foundation) or provide research support to a local hospital or university (e.g., Children's Cancer Research Fund of the University of Minnesota). Some disease-specific foundations also have small research portfolios devoted to children's cancer (e.g., Children's Brain Tumor Foundation; the Leukemia and Lymphoma Society), but this re-

TABLE 8.3 Selected State Projects Supported Through Special Projects of Regional and National Significance (SPRANS) and Community Integrated Service Systems (CISS) Grants

State	Description of project
Children with special health needs projects	
Alaska	• Developing systems of specialty care in rural and remote Alaska
	• Integrating pathways between the medical home and early intervention system using a parent navigation system
California	• Developing of a seamless, integrated system of care
Kansas	• Building systems for children with special health care needs in child care settings
Minnesota	• Developing transition from school to work services for youth with disabilities
New York	• Developing guidelines and outcome indicators for asthma, spina bifida, and sickle cell disease for managed care providers
Oklahoma	• Developing systems for children with special health needs and their families
Oregon	• Promoting partnerships between families of children with special health care needs and managed care plans
Vermont	• Implementing changes in the education and practice of families and professionals
Hemophilia and sickle cell disease projects	
Alabama	• Development of a statewide regionalized pediatric care system for individuals with hemoglobinopathies
Iowa	• Ensuring that a full range of services exist for adolescent and young adult patients with congenital bleeding disorders
Louisiana	• Providing for transition to adult care for adolescent sickle cell patients
North Carolina	• Providing comprehensive services for individuals with hemophilia and their families
Texas	• Providing comprehensive services, including medical and psychosocial services, for persons with hemophilia and related bleeding disorders, and for all complications of the disease
Traumatic brain injury (TBI) projects	
Arizona	• Developing a continuum of care for children with TBI and their families
Florida	• Enhancing the continuum of care and long-term supports for individuals with TBI through the development of interagency linkages and partnerships
Missouri	• Developing a comprehensive community-based program to meet the needs of individuals with TBI
Nevada	• Updating and implementing a statewide action plan to ensure a comprehensive community-based system of care

SOURCE: Health Resources and Services Administration, 2000a.

search is devoted almost exclusively to basic and clinical research that does not have a focus on survivorship. St. Jude Children's Research Hospital, located in Memphis, Tennessee, sponsors research and treatment of pediatric cancer, but does not have an extramural research program (see a description of its services in Chapter 5). The National Childhood Cancer Foundation supports research of the Children's Oncology Group and awards fellowships to outstanding young physicians to encourage their research work in the field of pediatric oncology (*www.nccf.org/foundation/ fellowships.asp*, accessed March 25, 2003). Only national organizations with a research grant program were included in the Board's review.

American Cancer Society

The American Cancer Society (ACS) is a nationwide, community-based, voluntary health organization involved in research, education, advocacy, and service (*http://www.cancer.org/docroot/AA/AA_0.asp*, accessed March 25, 2003). The ACS's overall annual expenditure in research was more than $130 million in Fiscal Year 2001, which includes extramural grants, intramural epidemiology and surveillance research, and an intramural behavioral research center. The extramural research program focuses primarily on peer-reviewed projects initiated by beginning investigators working in leading medical and scientific institutions.

A review of the ACS portfolio of extramural grants suggests that a total of $1.5 million was spent on four research projects related to pediatric cancer survivorship (Cheri Richard, Research Program Analyst, American Cancer Society, personal communication to Maria Hewitt, April 5, 2002):

- The Impact of Medical Treatment on the Quality of Life of Childhood Cancer Survivors: A Case Controlled Study
- Validation Testing of a New Brain-specific Measure for Pediatric Cancer Patients and Survivors
- Quality of Life in Children Who Survived Neuroblastoma
- Health Profiles in Adolescent Childhood Cancer Survivors

Lance Armstrong Foundation

Founded in 1997 by Lance Armstrong, the cancer survivor and four-time winner of the Tour de France bicycle race, the foundation bearing his name focuses on enhancing the quality of survival through support of survivor resources and support, groundbreaking survivorship programs, national advocacy initiatives, and scientific and clinical research grants (*www.laf.org*, accessed June 12, 2002). In 2000 and 2001 the foundation supported the following research activities:

- Promoting Health Behaviors Among Pediatric Cancer Survivors,
- Psychosocial, Behavioral and Pain Outcomes in Long-term Survivors of Childhood Cancer,
- A Pilot Intervention to Enhance Psychosexual Development in Adolescents and Young Adults with Cancer,
- Developing a Standardized Psychological Screening Tool for Childhood Cancer Survivors, and
- Pilot Test of an Intervention to Reduce Post-traumatic Stress in Young Adult Survivors of Childhood Cancer.

The foundations program and community care grants included:

- Life After Cancer Program at Cook Children's Medical Center,
- Living Well After Cancer Program at the University of Pennsylvania, and
- Wonders and Worries, Inc., a non-profit organization dedicated to providing psychological support for children, youth, and families coping with chronic life threatening illness.

RESEARCH PRIORITIES

Several priority areas for research emerged from the Board's review of childhood cancer survivorship research activities:

Assess the prevalence and etiology of late effects

- Support prospective longitudinal studies
- Develop a national childhood cancer registry from which cohorts could be selected (e.g., through the cooperation of existing population-based registries)
- Invest in infrastructure to improve capacity for long-term follow-up (e.g., systems to maintain current addresses)
- Advance methods to ensure maintenance of representative cohorts (e.g., minimize loss to follow-up)
- Standardize exposure and outcome measures (late effects, quality of life)

Test the potential for the reduction of late effects during treatment

- Expand support for clinical trials specifically designed to test the reduction of late effects with modifications of existing therapies

- Expand support for research on the substitution of current therapies with those likely to cause far less toxicity[3]

Develop interventions to prevent or reduce late effects after treatment

- Assess counseling and other interventions to mitigate long-term psychosocial effects of cancer and its treatment on individuals and their families
- Develop screening tests to identify those at high risk (e.g., early detection of impending ovarian failure)
- Evaluate the effectiveness of preventive health interventions (e.g., smoking cessation counseling, cancer screening regimens)
- Test chemoprevention strategies in this unique high-risk population.

Further improve quality of care to ameliorate the consequences of late effects on individuals and families

- Identify appropriate components of follow-up care through systematic evidence reviews, health services research, and consultation with patients and their families
- Identify optimal methods of delivering follow-up care through demonstration projects
- Develop screening tools to help determine who might benefit from psychosocial and other support services. Determine the optimal timing, frequency, and duration of interventions
- Identify models to facilitate reintegration into school or work following cancer treatment
- Assess the unique needs of medically underserved groups (minority populations) or populations (geographic areas)
- Evaluate methods to improve the education and training of health care providers

Investments in education and training are needed to further research. Examples of actions that could help expand the body of research in this area include: increased support for targeted fellowship programs in survivorship research, training and career development awards, center grants, visiting professorships, and the creation of special interest groups at academic meetings.

---

[3]The National Cancer Policy Board has a study in progress that will recommend ways to improve the process for developing better treatments for cancer, including a special focus on pediatric cancers (*www.IOM.edu/ncpb*).

SUMMARY AND CONCLUSIONS

There is a growing recognition that only through continued, systematic follow-up of large cohorts of survivors will the full extent of late effects be known. Amelioration of these late effects will require investments in intervention research. Ultimately, clinical research to find targeted therapies that maximize survival while minimizing late effects will likely improve the outlook for future generations of childhood cancer survivors. In the meantime, research is needed to optimize the recovery of cancer survivors and to test ways of delivering appropriate clinical and supportive care services.

Several ongoing research activities will answer many outstanding questions about late effects among childhood cancer survivors. The Childhood Cancer Survivor Study, in particular, will provide many opportunities for researchers. Relatively little multi-institutional survivorship research has taken place within the member institutions of the Children's Oncology Group, even though the majority of children with cancer receive their care in these settings. A renewed commitment to such research, along with investments in infrastructure to improve the ability to systematically identify and follow patients, would greatly improve the capacity and opportunities for survivorship research. While clinical, epidemiologic, and behavioral research in childhood survivorship has emerged to provide insights into childhood cancer survivorship, there appears to have been relatively little health services research to understand the health care experience and needs of childhood cancer survivors and their families.

REFERENCES

Bhatia S, Robison LL, Oberlin O, Greenberg M, Bunin G, Fossati-Bellani F, Meadows AT. 1996. Breast cancer and other second neoplasms after childhood Hodgkin's disease. *N Engl J Med* 334(12):745-51.

Bhatia S. 2002. Children's Oncology Group Late Effects Committtee. *National Cancer Policy Board Meeting*. Washington, DC.

Castleberry RP. 1997. Biology and treatment of neuroblastoma. *Pediatr Clin North Am* 44(4):919-37.

Children's Oncology Group. 2001. Requirements for Institutional Membership. Arcadia, CA: COG.

Health Resources and Services Administration . 2000a. *Title V: A Snapshot of Maternal and Child Health, 2000*. Rockville, MD: Health Resources and Services Administration.

Health Resources and Services Administration. 2000b. *Understanding Title V of the Social Security Act*. Rockville, MD: Health Resources and Services Aministration, The Maternal and Child Health Bureau.

Link, MP, Shuster JJ, Donaldson SS, Berard CW, Murphy SB. 1997. Treatment of children and young adults with early-stage non-Hodgkin's lymphoma. N Engl J Med. Oct 30; 337(18):1259-66.

Meadows AT, D'Angio GJ. 1974. Late effects of cancer treatment: methods and techniques for detection. *Semin Oncol* 1(1):87-90.

Meadows AT, Evans AE. 1976. Effects of chemotherapy on the central nervous system. A study of parenteral methotrexate in long-term survivors of leukemia and lymphoma in childhood. *Cancer* 37(2 Suppl):1079-85.

Meadows AT, D'Angio GJ, Evans AE, Harris CC, Miller RW, Mike V. 1975. Oncogenesis and other late effects of cancer treatment in children. *Radiology* 114(1):175-80.

National Cancer Institute. 1999. NCI Press Release: Cancer Survivorship. National Cancer Institute. Bethesda, MD: National Institutes of Health.

National Cancer Institute. National Cancer Institute. 2002a. *News from the NCI*. National Cancer Institute Research on Childhood Cancers. Bethesda, MD: National Institutes of Health (January 10, 2002).

National Cancer Institute. 2002b. *Office of Cancer Survivorship Factsheet*. Bethesda, MD: National Institutes of Health.

National Cancer Institute. 2002c. *The Nation's Investment in Cancer Research: A Plan and Budget Proposal for Fiscal Year 2004*. Bethesda, MD: National Institutes of Health.

Raney RB, Anderson JR, Barr FG, Donaldson SS, Pappo AS, Qualman SJ, Wiener ES, Maurer HM, Crist WM. 2001. Rhabdomyosarcoma and undifferentiated sarcoma in the first two decades of life: a selective review of intergroup rhabdomyosarcoma study group experience and rationale for Intergroup Rhabdomyosarcoma Study V. *J Pediatr Hematol Oncol* 23(4):215-20.

Robison LL, Mertens AC, Boice JD, Breslow NE, Donaldson SS, Green DM, Li FP, Meadows AT, Mulvihill JJ, Neglia JP, Nesbit ME, Packer RJ, Potter JD, Sklar CA, Smith MA, Stovall M, Strong LC, Yasui Y, Zeltzer LK. 2002. Study design and cohort characteristics of the Childhood Cancer Survivor Study: a multi-institutional collaborative project. *Med Pediatr Oncol* 38(4):229-39.

Shochat SJ, Fremgen AM, Murphy SB, Hutchison C, Donaldson SS, Haase GM, Provisor AJ, Clive-Bumpus RE, Winchester DP. 2001. Childhood cancer: patterns of protocol participation in a national survey. *CA Cancer J Clin* 51(2):119-30.

Smith M, Arthur D, Camitta B, Carroll AJ, Crist W, Gaynon P, Gelber R, Heerema N, Korn EL, Link M, Murphy S, Pui CH, Pullen J, Reamon G, Sallan SE, Sather H, Shuster J, Simon R, Trigg M, Tubergen D, Uckun F, Ungerleider R. 1996. Uniform approach to risk classification and treatment assignment for children with acute lymphoblastic leukemia. *J Clin Oncol* 14(1):18-24.

9

Findings and Recommendations

In this report, the Board has attempted to characterize the medical and psychosocial consequences of surviving childhood cancer, identify essential elements of quality care, explore some of the social and economic consequences facing cancer survivors such as under-insurance and employment discrimination, assess the status of applied clinical and health services research, and propose policies to improve the quality of care and quality of life for childhood cancer survivors and their families. This chapter summarizes the report's findings and presents recommendations (in order of their priority) to improve the health care and quality of life of survivors of childhood cancer.

Childhood cancer is rare, but with improvements in treatment over the past four decades, the size of the survivor population has grown dramatically. Five-year survival rates vary by type of childhood cancer, but overall, 78 percent of children diagnosed with cancer can expect to be alive in 5 years (Ries et al., 2002). In 1997, there were an estimated 270,000 survivors of childhood cancer, 95,000 of whom were under age 20 with the remainder being adults. This means that 1 in 810 individuals under age 20 have a history of cancer, and that 1 in 640 adults age 20 to 39 also have a history of childhood cancer.

Childhood cancers are a diverse set of diseases and the treatment of different types of cancer varies considerably. And within each type of cancer, the intensity and approach of treatment may differ depending on the child's age, general health, and characteristics of the cancer. The mainstays of cancer treatment are chemotherapy, radiation, and surgery. Most children are treated with two or three of these modalities, each of which can result in treatment-related health problems. Treatment of childhood cancer often occurs during important periods of physical, developmental, and psychological development. Complications, disabilities, or adverse outcomes that are the result of the disease process, the treatment, or both, are generally referred to as "late effects." Patterns of late effects have emerged among subgroups of childhood cancer survivors, which has contributed to an appreciation of cancer as a chronic disease with implications for long-term care.

As many as two-thirds of childhood cancer survivors are likely to experience at least one late effect, with perhaps one-fourth of survivors experiencing a late effect that is severe or life threatening. The most common late effects of childhood cancer are neurocognitive and psychological, cardiopulmonary, endocrine (e.g., those affecting growth and fertility), musculoskeletal, and related to second malignancies. The emergence of late effects depends on many factors, including age at diagnosis and treatment, exposures to chemotherapy and radiation during treatment (doses and parts of body exposed), and the severity of disease. Complicating the management of late effects is their variable nature. Some late effects are identified early in follow-up—during childhood or adolescent years—and resolve without consequence. Others may persist or develop in adulthood to become chronic problems or influence the progression of other diseases associated with aging. Understanding late effects is further complicated by the constant evolution of treatments. Cohorts of patients, representing different treatment eras, may experience unique sets of late effects. Some survivors of childhood cancer have positive psychosocial outcomes and there is a growing interest in better understanding resiliency among survivors.

DEVELOPING GUIDELINES FOR CARE

Recognizing the serious consequences of late effects, professional organizations and advocacy groups have recommended that an organized system of care be in place to address them. While there is general agreement that systematic follow-up should occur, there is no consensus regarding where such care should take place, who should provide it, its duration, and what the actual components of care should be.

Some aspects of follow-up care are understood to be necessary in most cases, though they may not be implemented. These include surveillance for recurrence of the original cancer or the development of a new cancer, assessing the psychosocial needs of survivors and their families, monitoring growth and maturation, counseling regarding preventive health, and testing for specific risk factors (e.g., exposure to hepatitis C following blood transfusions) or late effects (e.g., heart abnormalities, cognitive dysfunction, fertility impairment). Not well understood, however, is the optimal periodicity of follow-up contact, the value of specific screening/monitoring tests, and the effectiveness of interventions to ameliorate some late effects. Follow-up protocols are available, but they have generally been developed by individual institutions and vary in their recommendations. The lack of clarity regarding the effectiveness of interventions contributes to problems with health insurance reimbursement.

Clinical practice guidelines are "systematically developed statements to assist practitioner and patient decisions about appropriate health care for specific clinical circumstances" (Institute of Medicine, 1992). The foundation of clinical practice guidelines is a systematic review of available evidence—a scientific investigation that synthesizes the results of multiple primary investigations. Conducting a systematic review to answer a specific clinical questions general involves four steps (Cook et al., 1997; Institute of Medicine 2001):

1. a comprehensive search of potentially relevant articles using explicit, reproducible criteria in the selection of articles for review,
2. a critical appraisal of the scientific soundness of the research designs of the primary studies,
3. synthesis of data, and
4. interpretation of results.

To conduct systematic reviews, the Agency for Healthcare Research and Quality (AHRQ) supports 13 Evidence-Based Practice Centers (EPCs) in partnership with private-sector organizations (*http://www.ahcpr.gov/clinic/epcII.htm*, accessed March 17, 2003). Since 1997, the EPCs have completed 64 evidence reports, but none of them directly address issues related to survivors of childhood cancer.[1] The Late Effects Committee of the Children's Oncology Group (COG) has taken steps to develop guidelines for the follow-up of childhood cancer survivors (Melissa Hudson, St. Jude Children's Research Hospital, personal communication to Maria Hewitt, December 20, 2002). Guideline development requires considerable resources for conducting systematic reviews and for the full complement of needed expertise (e.g., health care providers, methodologists, consumers). The development and dissemination of guidelines alone has minimal effect on clinical practice, but a growing body of evidence indicates that guidelines implemented with systems in place to give providers information about

---

[1] One EPC report reviews evidence regarding the management of cancer-related pain, depression, and fatigue (*http://www.ahcpr.gov/clinic/epcsums/csympsum.htm*).

their practice and remind them of the guidelines can improve the quality of care. Up-front involvement of leaders from the health professions and representatives of patients in the guideline development process is also essential to guideline implementation (Institute of Medicine, 2001).

Recommendation 1: Develop evidence-based clinical practice guidelines for the care of survivors of childhood cancer.

The National Cancer Institute should convene an expert group of consumers, providers, and researchers to review available clinical practice guidelines and agree upon an evidence-based standard for current practice. For areas where bodies of evidence have not been rigorously evaluated, the Agency for Healthcare Research and Quality (AHRQ) Evidence Practice Centers (EPCs) should be charged to review the evidence. When evidence upon which to make recommendations is not available, the expert group should identify areas in need of research.

DESIGNING SYSTEMS OF CARE RESPONSIVE TO SURVIVORS' HEALTH CARE NEEDS

In some ways, the follow-up of survivors of childhood cancer is made easier by the extent to which children with cancer are treated in specialized centers of care. As many as 50 to 60 percent of children with cancer are initially treated in specialized cancer centers, but only an estimated 40 to 45 percent are receiving follow-up care in specialized clinics. Institutions that are members of the National Cancer Institute-funded pediatric cooperative group, the COG, are required to have on-site follow-up programs, but relatively few of them appear to have comprehensive, multidisciplinary programs. The Board has developed a description of the functions of an ideal follow-up system for survivors of childhood cancer (see Chapter 5, Box 5.5), but a minimum set of standards is needed to guide institutions in their development of programs to meet the wide-ranging needs of childhood cancer survivors.

According to the Board's review, four supportive care components are especially important to address in follow-up programs: 1) services to address the psychological implications of cancer to survivors and their families; 2) educational support through school transition programs; 3) personnel available to assist with issues related to insurance and employment problems; and 4) a plan to facilitate the transition of grown survivors of childhood cancer into adult systems of care.

Psychosocial Services

Despite periods of intense stress, most survivors achieve normal levels of psychological and social functioning, and families adapt well. All survivors, however, even those apparently doing quite well, experience at least occasional problems in social adjustment and continue to be concerned about their medical and social futures. In addition, there is a small but significant minority of survivors who remain seriously troubled and are impaired by their psychological problems. Some studies have demonstrated symptoms of post- traumatic stress disorder (PTSD) among survivors of childhood cancer, their siblings, and their parents, which signals a need to address the needs of entire families. Other research suggests that depression and anxiety may develop in response to poor academic achievement, secondary to late effects.

Psychosocial interventions to address these concerns can include psychological, emotional, peer, or education support; social skills training; adjustment counseling; family counseling; therapeutic play; cognitive-behavioral interventions; and group or individual psychoteherapy (Cohen and Walco, 1999; Kazak et al., 1999; Schwartz et al., 1999; Van Dongen-Melman, 2000; Walker, 1989). Personnel who can conduct routine assessments of need for these services and who are able to provide care or make appropriate referrals for care should be integral members of a follow-up system. At the same time, applied research is needed to better identify those survivors and their families who are most likely to benefit from psychosocial services, and the relative success of different types of interventions in improving quality of life. Some survivors cope well following their cancer treatment and report positive outcomes such as an increased appreciation of life. An improved understanding of how individuals and families adapt and remain resilient in the face of adversity can inform programs aimed at helping those individuals who are distressed.

Educational Services

School-related disabilities among survivors of childhood cancer may include learning disabilities and functional limitations. There are no good estimates of how many childhood cancer survivors need accommodations at school, but among certain groups of survivors, the need appears to be very high. There is, for example, a three- to fourfold increase in use of special education services among survivors of acute lymphocytic leukemia (ALL). Survivors of CNS tumors also are at very high risk of neurocognitive late effects and learning problems. Even if survivors are asymptomatic at school re-entry, they may require monitoring for long-term neurocognitive deficits that can arise in the years following treatment. More needs to be learned of the educational needs of other groups of childhood cancer survivors and of the effectiveness of interventions designed to ameliorate the late effects of cancer and its treatment.

Federal laws protect the educational rights of individuals with disabilities (i.e., the Individuals with Disabilities Education Act, the Rehabilitation Act of 1973, and the Americans with Disabilites Act). While legal protections appear to be comprehensive, procedures are implemented and laws are interpreted locally. Among parents, satisfaction with accommodations at schools varies depending on the school's level of cooperation, awareness of cognitive impairment in children with cancer, and resources available to provide the necessary interventions.

Given the central importance that school plays in a child's life, systems must be in place to assure an appropriate education following cancer treatment. Many cancer centers have transition programs to ease the return of childhood cancer survivors to school following their treatment. Ideally, planning for school re-entry begins at diagnosis and involves a school liaison to ensure that educational environments are supportive and can accommodate any late effects. School systems are generally not familiar with the particular needs of cancer survivors and may not support all services needed by childhood cancer survivors returning (or going) to school. Repeated neuropsychologic assessments may, for example, be necessary to gauge educational needs and progress, and yet are routinely excluded from coverage by federally mandated special education programs. Such testing may also be difficult to obtain through private insurance plans (see Chapter 7). A cancer center-based school liaison can play an important role in advocating for children as they re-enter school and can monitor the educational progress of survivors through transitions to college, employment, or vocational programs.

Employment- and Insurance-Related Protections

Significant progress has been made since the early 1990s to improve the employment opportunities of cancer survivors. With the passage of federal laws such as the Americans with Disabilities Act and the Family and Medical Leave Act, as well as the expansion of many state laws, cancer survivors have gained new legal rights and remedies. Additionally, the rise of cancer survivorship advocacy has helped dispel the myths that fuel survivors' employment problems. While employment discrimination has declined over time, problems appear to have persisted for some survivors of childhood cancer.

Providing better information to survivors regarding employment rights may lessen the effects of cancer on employment opportunities. All working-aged (or near working-age) survivors should receive from their cancer center and/or oncologist information about their legal rights, including information on how to avoid employment problems and how to respond to employment discrimination. Additionally, everyone who provides psychosocial support (such as oncology nurses, social workers, psychologists, counselors, and peer support organizations) should be familiar with cancer survivors' rights. Health care providers can further help their patients avoid job problems by educating employers about their patients' prognoses, abilities, and limitations and assist in the identification of reasonable accommodations.

Transition from Pediatric to Adult Systems of Care

Roughly one-third of newly diagnosed children with cancer are adolescents age 15 to 19. While most adolescents are treated by pediatric oncologists, they likely transition to adult care providers within a few years of completing therapy. Those under age 15 would be expected to remain in pediatric care for a longer period, but they and their families would need to have a plan for continued care as young adults. The American Academy of Pediatrics and the American Academy of Family Physicians, the American College of Physicians, and the American Society of Internal Medicine have addressed the issue of transition care for young adults with special health care needs and have recommended several steps to achieve appropriate transition from pediatric health care to adults health care (Box 9.1) (American Academy of Pediatrics, 2002; Kelly et al., 2002; Reiss and Gibson, 2002; Scal, 2002). The Board considered these recommendations relevant to pediatric oncology providers and endorses them. Of particular interest to the Board was the concept of partnership and the comanagement of care for a period of time. As applied in the context of survivorship care, this would allow pediatric oncologists to work with adult primary care practitioners, allowing them to become familiar with issues of late effects and their management while at the same time assuring continuity of care. A portable and accessible medical summary that can provide a common knowledge base for collaboration among health care providers is also critical to a successful transition to adult care.

A number of approaches have been proposed to address the needs of childhood cancer survivors, from follow-up clinics located in cancer centers to a national virtual consultation service organized through the internet. For many survivors and their families, geographic distance from a cancer center precludes easy access to follow-up. Most survivors are in contact with primary care providers, but the extent to which cancer-related issues are addressed in this context is not known. Few examples of collaborative practice, an approach that relies on a planned working together of oncology providers and primary care physicians, have been described. Such a

---

Box 9.1
Critical First Steps to Ensuring Successful Transitioning to Adult-Oriented Health Care

1. Ensure that all young people with special health care needs have an identified health care professional who attends to the unique challenges of transition and assumes responsibility for current health care, care coordination, and future health care planning. This responsibility is executed in partnership with other child and adult health care professionals, the young person, and his or her family. It is intended to ensure that as transitions occur, all young people have uninterrupted, comprehensive, and accessible care within their community.

2. Identify the core knowledge and skills required to provide developmentally appropriate health care transition services to young people with special health care needs and make them part of training and certification requirements for primary care residents and physicians in practice.

3. Prepare and maintain an up-to-date medical summary that is portable and accessible. This information is critical for successful health care transition and provides the common knowledge base for collaboration among health care professionals.

4. Create a written health care transition plan by age 14 together with the young person and family. At a minimum, this plan should include what services need to be provided, who will provide them, and how they will be financed. This plan should be reviewed and updated annually and whenever there is a transfer of care.

5. Apply the same guidelines for primary and preventive care for all adolescents and young adults, including those with special health care needs, recognizing that young people with special health care needs may require more resources and services than do other young people to optimize their health.

6. Ensure affordable, continuous health insurance coverage for all young people with special health care needs throughout adolescence and adulthood. This insurance should cover appropriate compensation for 1) health care transition planning for all young people with special health care needs, and 2) care coordination for those who have complex medical conditions.

SOURCE: American Academy of Pediatrics, 2002.

---

model could facilitate the necessary transition from pediatric-based care to adult care as childhood cancer survivors mature into adulthood. Cancer survivors, while having some unique needs, are similar to survivors of other chronic illness. There are likely opportunities to develop efficient systems of care to address at least some of the needs of individuals with a broad range of chronic illnesses and conditions. Survivors of childhood cancer with neurocognitive impairment, for example, share medical and long-term care needs with children who have brain injuries and other neurologic conditions. Such children may be followed by a neurologist, but often do not have easy access to support services needed to accommodate adjustment to school, work, or independent living.

There is little evidence to suggest that any particular mechanism is optimal for delivering follow-up care to survivors of childhood cancer. Rather than recommending any one approach, the Board felt that agreement is needed on what constitutes the essential elements of follow-up care. Demonstration programs with rigorous evaluations are then needed to test the merits of alternative methods to deliver these elements of care.

> *Recommendation 2: Define a minimum set of standards for systems of comprehensive, multidisciplinary follow-up care that link specialty and primary care providers, ensure the presence of such a system within institutions treating children with cancer, and evaluate alternate models of delivery of survivorship care.*

• The National Cancer Institute (NCI) should convene an expert group of consumers, providers, and health services researchers to define essential components of a follow-up system and propose alternative ways to deliver care. Consideration could be given to long-term follow-up clinics, collaborative practices between oncology and primary care physicians, and other models that might be dictated by local practices and resources, patient and family preferences, geography, and other considerations. Any system that is developed should assure linkages between specialty and primary care providers.

• A set of minimal standards for designation as a late effects clinic should be endorsed and adopted by relevant bodies such as COG, the American Society of Pediatric Hematology/Oncology, the American Academy of Pediatrics, the American Society of Clinical Oncology, the American College of Surgeons' Commission on Cancer, and NCI in its requirements for approval for comprehensive cancer centers.

• COG members and other institutions treating children with cancer should ensure that a comprehensive, multidisciplinary system of follow-up care is in place to serve the needs of patients and their families discharged from their care.

• State comprehensive cancer control plans being developed and implemented with CDC support should include provisions to ensure appropriate follow-up care for cancer survivors and their families.

• Grant programs of the Health Resources and Services Administration (e.g., Special Projects of Regional and National Significance [SPRANS]) should support demonstration programs to test alternate delivery systems (e.g., telemedicine, outreach programs) to ensure that the needs of different populations are met (e.g., rural residents or those living far from specialized late-effects clinics, ethnic and minority groups). Needed also are evaluations to determine which models of care confer benefits in terms of preventing or ameliorating late effects and improving quality of life, and which models survivors and their families prefer.

RAISING SURVIVORS' AWARENESS OF LATE EFFECTS

Recent research shows that the majority of cancer survivors appear to be unaware of their risk for late effects or the need for follow-up care. They also lack specific information regarding their disease history and treatment that would be needed by a clinician to provide appropriate follow-up care. The reasons why survivors lack knowledge about late effects is not known. In the case of older survivors, this lack of knowledge could be explained if care was completed before the full scope of late effects associated with their cancer and its treatment were known. If parents of survivors treated at very young ages had received information on late effects, they may not have retained or effectively communicated that information to their child. Parents of low socioeconomic status, who do not speak English, or who face cultural barriers, may have greater difficulty in this regard. Anecdotal evidence from parents and survivors suggests that late effects have not been routinely addressed by pediatric oncologists (Nancy Keene, personal communication to Maria Hewitt, December 21, 2001)

Effective interventions are available to prevent or ameliorate some late effects and a failure to receive appropriate follow-up care can be life threatening and compromise quality of life.

Recommendation 3: Improve awareness of late effects and their implications to long-term health among childhood cancer survivors and their families.

- Clinicians providing pediatric cancer care should provide survivors and their families written information regarding the specific nature of their cancer and its treatment, the risks of late effects, and a plan (and when appropriate, referrals) for follow-up. Discussions of late effects should begin with diagnosis.
- Public and private sponsors of health education (e.g., NCI, American Cancer Society) should launch informational campaigns and provide support to survivorship groups that have effective outreach programs.

AUGMENTING PROFESSIONAL EDUCATION AND TRAINING

If survivorship care is to expand and improve, additional professional education and training opportunities will be needed. Advance practice pediatric oncology nurses have provided leadership in establishing and managing survivorship clinics, but there are relatively few such trained nurses and the oncology content in most nursing training programs is limited (Ettinger, 2002). Oncologists who completed their training more than a decade ago may not be familiar with the full scope of late effects now recognized. And given the cursory coverage of survivorship issues in medical texts and curricula, there is a need for continuing medical education and other educational opportunities for oncologists. A model for continuing education for primary care providers is a home study self-assessment monograph developed by the American Academy of Family Physicians on adult survivorship issues (Hamblin, 2002). Shortcomings in training of other personnel who might practice within a follow-up care system (e.g., psychologists, oncology social workers) also need to be addressed. About 1 in 300 ambulatory care visits among children and adolescents is cancer related. As the number of childhood cancer survivors increases, primary care providers will encounter childhood cancer survivors in their practices more often. However, these providers may miss opportunities to intervene to ameliorate late effects because they have little experience with childhood cancer survivors and lack training. Primary care providers learn about cancer in their training and in their practice, and that knowledge should be extended to include late effects. Knowing who to contact for assistance when questions arise regarding the management of the late effects of cancer and its treatment is also valuable.

Recommendation 4: Improve professional education and training regarding late effects of childhood cancer and their management for both specialty and primary care providers.

• Professional societies should act to improve primary care providers' awareness through professional journals, meetings, and continuing education opportunities.
• Primary care training programs should include information about the late effects of cancer in their curriculum.
• NCI should provide easy-to-find information on late effects of childhood cancer on its website (e.g., through the Physician Data Query [PDQ], which provides up-to-date information on cancer prevention, treatment, and supportive care).
• Oncology training programs should organize coursework, clinical

practicums, and continuing education programs on late effects of cancer treatment for physicians, nurses, social workers, and other providers.

• Oncology professional organizations should, if they have not already, organize committees or subcommittees dedicated to issues related to late effects.

• Oncology Board examinations should include questions related to late effects of cancer treatment.

• Interdisciplinary professional meetings that focus on the management of late effects should be supported to raise awareness of late effects among providers who may encounter childhood cancer survivors in their practices (e.g., cardiologists, neurologists, fertility specialists, psychologists).

STRENGTHENING PUBLIC PROGRAMS SERVING CHILDHOOD CANCER SURVIVORS

Some of the concerns of childhood cancer survivors are unique to their cancer and its treatment. However, the concerns of many survivors experiencing late effects are shared by children and young adults with other chronic illnesses and disabling conditions. Several of the key public programs that serve such children could be strengthened to assure that cancer survivors receive supportive care. These programs are housed in the U.S. Department of Health and Human Services (DHHS) and in the U.S. Department of Education (DOE). Coordination among public programs serving children and young adults is generally poor. There are differing eligibility criteria, covered services, and relationships among federal, state, and local partners. No one program has a specific mission to address the special needs of survivors of childhood cancers or to provide the full spectrum of services these children need.

As part of the DHHS Healthy People 2010 initiative, the Maternal and Child Health Bureau in the Health Resources and Services Administration (HRSA) and key partners (e.g., provider and consumer groups) have launched an effort to assure that the needs of families across the nation are met. Progress toward meeting the needs of children with special health care need is being measured with the following set of core program objectives (Department of Health and Human Services, 2001):

1. All children with special health care needs will receive coordinated, ongoing comprehensive care within a medical home.

2. All families of children with special health care needs will have adequate private and/or public insurance to pay for the services they need.

3. All children will be screened early and continuously for special health care needs.

4. Families of children with special health care needs will partner in decision making at all levels and will be satisfied with the services they receive.

5. Community-based service system will be organized so families can use them easily.

6. All youth with special health care needs will receive the services necessary to make transitions to all aspects of adult life, including adult health care, work and independence.

The public programs available to help accomplish these important goals include:

1. The Maternal and Child Health Block Grant and its program for Children with Special Health Care Needs (DHHS/HRSA)

2. The Medicaid Program (DHHS/Centers for Medicare and Medicaid Services [CMS])

3. The State Children's Health Insurance Program (S-CHIP: DHHS/ CMS)

4. The Bureau of Primary Health Care, its network of community health centers, and its supported health care professional workforce (DHHS/ HRSA)

5. The Early Intervention Program (DOE)

6. Special Education Programs for Individuals with Disabilities (DOE)

All of these federal programs operate in partnership with state and local governments. Each program has its own eligibility requirements, which may be based on health-related criteria and/or income and assets.

Each state has a Program for Children with Special Health Care Needs (CSHCN), funded in part through the Maternal and Child Health Block Grant. The program provides health and support services to children "who have, or are at increased risk for, chronic physical, developmental, behavioral, or emotional conditions and who also require health and related services of a type or amount beyond that required by children generally" (*www.mchb.hrsa.gov*, accessed March 7, 2003). In 1989, Congress amended the Maternal and Child Health Block Grant authorization to require state CSHCN programs "to provide and to promote family-centered, community-based, coordinated care (including care coordination services . . .) for children with special health care needs . . ." and to "facilitate the development of community-based systems of services for such children and their families" (Gittler, undated). State CSHCN programs now offer training, finance community support organizations, and promote policies to further coordination of care and communication. These safety net programs have the potential to extend supportive services to survivors of childhood cancer and to provide links between highly specialized care and primary care for these children. State programs, however, currently provide an inconsistent level of services and have varying eligibility criteria that may exclude survivors of childhood cancer. States coordinate their CSHCN, Medicaid, and S-CHIP programs, but the degree and purposes of coordination differ. Medical and support services should be coordinated among federal, state, and local programs.

To meet the goals of continuous monitoring for special health care needs, and particularly to ensure that survivors of childhood cancer have a medical home, much stronger systems of care are needed. Education of both community-based primary care providers and cancer center-based specialists about the needs of these children and their families is essential. Simpler communication systems that assure prompt information-sharing among all those caring for these children must be established and supported, and must be responsive to family concerns and preferences. Eligibility and program requirements that create gaps in services and restrict access to appropriate care and support services by survivors of childhood cancer must be changed. Capacity building that emphasizes the medical home, communication among primary care providers and specialists caring for and monitoring survivors of childhood cancer, and adequate support and educational services for these children is essential.

Recommendation 5: The Health Resources and Services Administration's Maternal and Child Health Bureau and its partners should be fully supported in implementing the Healthy People 2010 goals for Children with Special Health Care Needs. These efforts include a national communication strategy, efforts at capacity building, setting standards, and establishing accountability. Meeting these goals will benefit survivors of childhood cancer and other children with special health care needs.

IMPROVING ACCESS TO HEALTH CARE SERVICES

Ideally, all Americans, regardless of medical history or employment status, would have health insurance coverage and access to affordable, quality medical care. Broad-based national health insurance reform is unlikely to take place in the near future. Instead, cancer survivors' best hope for significant insurance reform rests with federal and state legislation that targets specific issues. Because federal legislation generally covers only federal programs, such as Medicare and Medicaid, many insurance reforms must be addressed at the state level. States could, for example, expand access to health insurance through increased support of state high-risk insurance pools. Such insurance pools provide coverage to individuals who have been denied private health insurance in the individual market. Roughly half of states have such programs and among those that do, the pools have had a limited impact in making insurance available and affordable to otherwise uninsurable individuals because of high premiums, deductibles, and copayments, and restricted annual and lifetime benefits (Achman and Chollet, 2001). A recent federal initiative helps states create high-risk pools to increase access to health coverage (DHHS press release, 2002). In the absence of major changes in the delivery and financing of U.S. health care, incremental reforms regarding particular benefits or improved patient protections must be considered carefully because when reforms increase the costs of insurance products, they can unintentionally increase rates of uninsuredness. The IOM's Committee on the Consequences of Uninsurance will consider selected programs and proposals involving insurance-based strategies to expand health insurance coverage (*www.iom.edu*) in the sixth in a series of reports that address problems related to uninsurance.

Despite state efforts to reduce the number of uninsured children through S-CHIP, often through expansions of state Medicaid programs, many children remain uninsured. The Medicaid Program and S-CHIP insure more than one-quarter of American children, all of them living in families with low incomes. Many of the post-treatment services needed by survivors of childhood cancer with Medicaid coverage would be available through the Early and Periodic Screening, Diagnosis and Treatment (EPSDT) program. These Medicaid services are dictated by federal statute and include "diagnostic, screening, preventive, and rehabilitative services, including medical or remedial services recommended for the maximum reduction of physical or mental disability and restoration of an individual to the best possible functional level (in facility, home, or other setting)" (*http://www.healthlaw. org/pubs/19990323epsdtfact.html*, accessed March 9, 2003). In practice, several barriers to EPSDT have limited use of services, including a shortage of providers participating in the Medicaid program, beneficiaries who are not informed of the program and its benefits, and issues related to cost.

Many individuals insured privately or through the Medicaid program are enrolled in fully capitated managed care arrangements. Managed care plans may control the use of specialists, especially those practicing outside of their plans' networks. Some research suggests that the services and specialists needed by children and young adults with special health care needs are not always available within plans and their networks. Contracts between insurance purchasers (e.g., employers, state Medicaid officials) and health plans should ensure an appropriate complement of services and range of providers necessary to meet the needs of children with special health care needs. These requirements should be based on evidence of the effectiveness of services.

For individuals with inadequate insurance and financial resources, there is a patchwork of public and private programs for primary care. Full support of federally supported Community and Migrant Health Centers and other programs aimed at underserved groups enhances the nation's health care safety net.

Recommendation 6: Federal, state, and private efforts are needed to optimize childhood cancer survivors' access to appropriate resources and delivery systems through both health insurance reforms and support of safety net programs such as the Health Resources and Services Administration's Community and Migrant Health Centers.

INCREASING RESEARCH ON CHILDHOOD CANCER SURVIVORSHIP

Recognition is growing that only continued, systematic follow-up of large cohorts of survivors can reveal the full extent of late effects. Amelioration of these late effects will require investments in intervention research. Ultimately, clinical research to find targeted therapies that maximize survival while minimizing late effects will likely improve the outlook for future generations of childhood cancer survivors. In the meantime, research is needed to optimize the recovery of cancer survivors and to test ways of delivering appropriate clinical and supportive care services. This under-recognized area of research needs new support.

Several ongoing research activities will answer many outstanding questions about late effects among childhood cancer survivors. The Childhood Cancer Survivor Study, in particular, will provide many opportunities for researchers. Relatively little multi-institutional survivorship research has taken place within the member institutions of the Children's Oncology Group, even though the majority of children with cancer receive their care in these settings. A renewed commitment to such research, along with investments in infrastructure to improve the ability to systematically identify and follow patients, would greatly improve the capacity and opportunities for survivorship research. While clinical, epidemiologic, and behavioral research in childhood survivorship has emerged to provide insights into childhood cancer survivorship, there appears to have been relatively little health services research to understand the health care experience and needs of childhood cancer survivors and their families.

The need for survivorship follow-up care is widely acknowledged and general recommendations for such care are available to clinicians, survivors, and their families. An active research program is needed to address the many questions regarding the necessary components of follow-up care in the identification, prevention, and amelioration of specific late effects.

The Board recognized the following areas for needed research. (Detailed research priorities are outlined in Chapter 8.)

> *Recommendation 7: Public and private research organizations (e.g., NCI, National Institute of Nursing Research, American Cancer Society) should increase support for research to prevent or ameliorate the long-term consequences of childhood cancer. Priority areas of research include assessing the prevalence and etiology of late effects; testing methods that may reduce late effects during treatment; developing interventions to prevent or reduce late effects after treatment; and furthering improvements in quality of care to ameliorate the consequences of late effects on individuals and families.*

• Both prospective and retrospective studies are needed to quantify the incidence and prevalence of adverse sequelae in representative cohorts of survivors. Establishing a population-based surveillance system for childhood cancer would facilitate population-based research efforts.

• Studies are needed of new treatments to reduce the occurrence of late effects among childhood cancer survivors and of interventions designed to prevent or ameliorate the consequences of late effects associated with current treatments.

• Research is needed on the long-term social, economic, and quality of life implications of cancer on survivors and their families.

• The COG should be supported in adding long-term follow-up to its clinical trials. There is an obligation to evaluate late effects of therapeutic interventions under study. Prospective clinical assessments are needed to learn about late effects.

• The CCSS cohort study should be fully supported and researchers encouraged to use data that have been collected. Resources are needed to assure completeness of follow-up of survivors and to conduct methodologic studies (e.g., assessment of the adequacy of sibling controls for psychosocial and health outcomes).

• Opportunities to study late effects within systems of care that have a medical record system that captures primary and specialty care should be explored (e.g., through the HMO network, an NCI-supported research consortium of HMOs with population-based research program).

• As evidence emerges regarding late effects, research institutions should have systems in place to disseminate information to survivors who remain under their care, and to providers of follow-up care, in both specialty and primary care settings.

The National Cancer Policy Board has proposed a comprehensive policy agenda that links expansions in research, improvements in health care delivery, infrastructure development, survivor education, professional education and training, and assurances of coverage under federal insurance and service programs to improve the long-term outlook for the growing population of childhood cancer survivors.[2]

REFERENCES

Achman L, Chollet D. 2001. Insuring the Uninsurable: An Overview of State High-Risk Health Insurance Pools. Mathematica Policy Research, Inc. Princeton NJ (http://www.mathematica-mpr.com/3rdlevel/uninsurablehot.htm. Last accessed March 21, 2003).

American Academy of Pediatrics. 2002. A consensus statement on health care transitions for young adults with special health care needs. *Pediatrics* 110(6 Pt 2):1304-6.

Cohen SO, Walco GA. 1999. Dance/Movement therapy for children and adolescents with cancer. *Cancer Pract* 7(1):34-42.

Cook DJ, Mulrow CD, Haynes RB. 1997. Systematic reviews: synthesis of best evidence for clinical decisions. *Ann Intern Med* 126(5):376-80.

Department of Health and Human Services, Health Resources and Services Administration . 2001. *Achieving Success for All Children and Youth With Special Health Care Needs: A 10-Year Action Plan to Accompany Healthy People 2010.* Washington DC: US DHHS.

Department of Health and Human Services, CMS. 2002. HHS to Help States Create High-Risk Pools to Increase Access to Health Coverage. Press release, November 26, 2002. (www.hhs.gov/news/press/2002pres/20021126a.html, last accessed January 31, 2003).

Ettinger A. 2002. *Long-Term Survivor Programs: A Paradigm for the Advanced Practice Nurse.* NCPB Commissioned Paper.

Hamblin J.E., Schifeling D.E. 2002. *Cancer Survivors (Monograph 264).* American Academy of Family Practice.

Institute of Medicine, Committee on Clinical Practice Guidelines. 1992. Field MJ, Lohr KN. *Guidelines for Clinical Practice : From Development to Use.* Washington, D.C.: National Academy Press.

Institute of Medicine, Committee on Quality of Health Care in America. 2001. *Crossing the Quality Chasm: A New Health System for the 21st Century.* Washington, D.C.: National Academy Press.

Kazak AE, Simms S, Barakat L, Hobbie W, Foley B, Golomb V, Best M. 1999. Surviving cancer competently intervention program (SCCIP): a cognitive- behavioral and family therapy intervention for adolescent survivors of childhood cancer and their families. *Fam Process* 38(2):175-91.

Kelly AM, Kratz B, Bielski M, Rinehart PM. 2002. Implementing transitions for youth with complex chronic conditions using the medical home model. *Pediatrics* 110(6 Pt 2): 1322-7.

Meadows AT, Black B, Nesbit ME Jr, Strong LC, Nicholson HS, Green DM, Hays DM, Lozowski SL. 1993. Long-term survival. Clinical care, research, and education. *Cancer* 71(10 Suppl):3213-5.

---

[2]The Board's recommendations are consistent with those made by Meadows and colleagues following a workshop discussion on long-term survival in 1993 .

Reiss J, Gibson R. 2002. Health care transition: destinations unknown. *Pediatrics* 110(6 Pt 2):1307-14.

Ries LAG, Eisner MP, Kosary CL, Hankey BF, Miller BA, Clegg L, Edwards BK, Editors. 2002. *SEER Cancer Statistics Review, 1973-1999*. Bethesda, MD: National Cancer Institute.

Scal P. 2002. Transition for youth with chronic conditions: primary care physicians' approaches. *Pediatrics* 110(6 Pt 2):1315-21.

Schwartz CE, Feinberg RG, Jilinskaia E, Applegate JC. 1999. An evaluation of a psychosocial intervention for survivors of childhood cancer: paradoxical effects of response shift over time: *Psychooncology* 8(4):344-54.

Van Dongen-Melman JE. 2000. Developing psychosocial aftercare for children surviving cancer and their families. *Acta Oncol* 39(1):23-31.

Walker C. 1989. Use of art and play therapy in pediatric oncology. *J Pediatr Oncol Nurs* 6(4):121-6.